Hospital Infection Prevention

Chand Wattal • Nancy Khardori
Editors

Hospital Infection Prevention

Principles & Practices

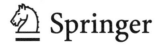 Springer

Editors
Chand Wattal
Clinical Microbiology and Immunology
Sir Ganga Ram Hospital
New Delhi, India

Nancy Khardori
Department of Internal Medicine
Eastern Virginia Medical School
Virginia, USA

ISBN 978-81-322-1607-0   ISBN 978-81-322-1608-7 (eBook)
DOI 10.1007/978-81-322-1608-7
Springer New Delhi Heidelberg New York Dordrecht London

Library of Congress Control Number: 2013952932

Printed on acid-free paper

Springer is part of Springer Science+Business Media (www.springer.com)

Foreword

I have had the privilege of reviewing "The Principles and Practices of Infection Prevention" edited by Dr. Nancy Khardori and Dr. Chand Wattal. This monograph has been carefully edited to provide a balanced view of important topics covered by various authors including the editors themselves. It provides an easy read for both veterans in infectious diseases and those getting introduced to this specialty as beginners. Editors note that this monograph focuses on "nonglamorous" field of infection prevention. While it may be a design to make the reading less threatening, it is no exaggeration that infection prevention is one of the most important functions of any healthcare facility particularly when there is a reflexive tendency to use antibiotics on slightest pretext.

Both editors have decades of cumulative experience to share with readers. Dr. Khardori has experience of nearly two decades serving as the Medical Director at University level besides also serving as the Medical Director for Infection Control for the state of Illinois. Dr. Khardori is a trained microbiologist as well as an internist with subspecialty training in infectious disease. She is board certified by the American Board of Internal Medicine in the subspecialty of infectious disease. Additionally she is qualified by the American Board of Microbiology.

Dr. Wattal is a physician and a trained microbiologist overseeing the department of microbiology at Sir Ganga Ram Hospital in New Delhi (India). He has been successful in creating a unique bench to bedside collaboration in his institution which makes the microbiology laboratory results very relevant to patient care. He has been overseeing and upgrading the infection control service at his institution and providing direction to a number of other institutions around the country. His efforts in infection control won his hospital the Hospital Management Asia award.

This monograph begins with an overview of microbial world focusing on various modes of transmission covering organisms such as bacteria, viruses, mycobacteria, fungi, protozoa, and worms. An entire chapter has been devoted to vaccination – the most important modality of infection prevention. This focus often gets a short shrift in many monographs devoted to infection control. Additionally this monograph provides review of hospital infection control programs and the associated processes highlighting role of hospital infection control committee, and its functionaries (epidemiologist, microbiologist, pharmacist, clinicians, and the all important – nursing staff). Given the editors' background in microbiology, it is not surprising to see a prominent section addressing the role of microbiology laboratory in infection prevention. A chapter has been devoted to "antimicrobial stewardship" which is critical to preventing/reducing emergence of antimicrobial resistance. This chapter addresses goals of antibiotic stewardship program including role of interdisciplinary team focusing on formulating and implementing policies and procedures in a very precise manner. A brief four-step process has been described.

Issues pertaining to housekeeping, disinfection, and waste management have been addressed in a very clear and user-friendly manner. Often this focus is wanting in many monographs of this kind. Processes of decontamination and sterilization have been discussed in appropriate detail. This section also covers the controversial issue of reuse of "single-use" medical devices providing much needed guidance in this area. Focus and emphasis on the importance of "hand hygiene" in infection prevention have been given its deserved place.

This text covers individual high-risk areas within the hospital that deserve special emphasis such as ICUs, dialysis units, operating suits, maternity suits, and burn units. There is a very effective section dealing with bloodstream infections and urinary tract infections pertaining to "open ward."

Overall, I believe the reader will find this monograph as an excellent resource and update pertaining to infection control programs and practices for both those entering the field of infection control and those already possessing expertise in this area.

Eastern Virginia Medical School   Edward C. Oldfield III
Sentara Norfolk General Hospital
Norfolk, VA, USA

Preface

"First do no harm" is the operating principle for physicians taking care of patients in a healthcare setting. This book addresses a potential unintended event that can occur while receiving healthcare and thus breach this fundamental trust. It is outrageous but commonplace to find a patient admitted for an elective surgery developing urinary tract infection just because a urinary catheter was placed to facilitate overall care. Unfortunately, the curriculum of medical graduates or even postgraduates in most of the universities is not adequate enough to impart knowledge on principles of infection prevention in day-to-day practice of medicine. Instead, they are expected to memorize a set of "Infection Control Guidelines." The misconception in the front lines is that these guidelines need to be adhered to simply to "stay out of trouble." Prevention of infection as the nonglamorous but an integral part of medical care needs to be understood rather than practiced with automation in order to get passion into the equation.

This monograph is aimed at blending principles and practices of infection prevention primarily in hospital settings but also addresses an important area of prevention, namely, using vaccines, usually ignored, has also been included for comprehensive reading. It is a paradox that India being the biggest vaccine producer for the rest of the world utilizes the same the least for its own population. The contributors to this monograph are directly involved in the efforts to reduce morbidity and mortality from hospital-acquired infections. The vast knowledge and hands-on experience in the principles and practices of infection prevention for decades are shared in a very reader-friendly manner. The introductory chapter "The Mighty World of Microbes" has tried to impress as to how extensive the world of microorganisms existing around us is and provides a rationale for understanding the principles behind practices of infection prevention. The various practices of infection prevention have already been laid down by various international bodies to allow an organized and consistent approach to the complex problem of hospital-acquired infections. A hospital infection prevention program along with an understanding of the role of medical microbiology laboratory and an active antibiotic stewardship program can go a long way in making healthcare facilities much safer than what they are in spite of major advances in managing serious illnesses. It is essential for prevention of hospital-acquired infections to understand and implement relevant policies with regard to disinfection and waste management by the hospital administrators. The concept of segregation of waste at the point of its generation has resulted in a sea change in the management and disposal of hospital waste. While this is being practiced by healthcare workers, it is the moral responsibility of the administrators to provide appropriate personal protective equipment and facilities especially for hand hygiene to prevent the healthcare personnel contracting the very diseases that they help their patients overcome. Often emphasis is laid on environmental monitoring, whereas enough evidence exists in literature as to where routine environmental surveillance is not recommended unless there is an outbreak-like scenario. This monograph has tried to address some of the controversial aspects of disinfection and sterilization and has tried to take those issues to a logical conclusion with evidence. It is essential to address in detail the disinfection and sterilization concepts that need to be pursued with zest and zeal in the high-risk areas and for procedures conducted on floor by the medical staff. The training of medical staff should start at the very outset of their professional career so that routine infection prevention practices can become "habit forming" if not addictive.

The creation and persistence of antibiotic-resistant bacteria has added a particularly dangerous dimension to the short falls in infection prevention. Since we are at the end of the road for search of newer antibiotics, it is the responsibility of the medical fraternity to preserve such precious and lifesaving reserves like antibiotics. Antibiotic stewardship practiced and accepted at the institutional level is hallmark of appropriate and long-lasting use of antibiotics. This monograph could not have been possible without the participation of all of its contributors who took upon themselves to share their experiences. Special thanks are owed to Dr. J. K. Oberoi for the time and understanding she has contributed to the successful completion of the first-of-its-kind monograph published in India.

New Delhi, India   Chand Wattal
Virginia, USA   Nancy Khardori

Contents

Part I

The Mighty World of Microbes:
An Overview

The Mighty World of Microbes: An Overview

Iass El Lakkis and Nancy Khardori

The Microbial World On and Around Us

The world of microbes on our planet is vast and diverse. This includes the normal bacterial flora present on the skin and mucous membranes of humans. The human microbiome project (HMP) was launched by NIH in 2007 as a part of a road map for medical research. The HMP serves as a template for researchers who are studying more than 1,000 microbial genomes with a focus on their role in health and disease. The study samples have been derived from five human body regions that are known to be inhabited by microbial flora. These include the gastrointestinal tract, female urogenital tract, mouth, nose, and skin. The techniques being used include finger printing, sequencing, dynamic range, and comparison of multiple samples. It is now well accepted that there are more microbial cells than human cells in the human body. Just the gastrointestinal tract harbors more than tenfold micro-

I. El Lakkis, M.D.
Division of Infectious Diseases, Department of Internal Medicine, Eastern Virginia Medical School, Norfolk, VA, USA

N. Khardori, M.D., Ph.D. (✉)
Division of Infectious Diseases, Department of Internal Medicine, Eastern Virginia Medical School, Norfolk, VA, USA

Department of Microbiology and Molecular Cell Biology, Eastern Virginia Medical School, Norfolk, VA, USA
e-mail: nkhardori@gmail.com

bial cells than the number of human cells in the entire body. The understanding of the relationship between microbes and humans is at best rudimentary at this point in time. Similarly, the relationship between humans and microbes in the environment and environmental surfaces is poorly understood except for a few pathogenic microbes.

The most well-studied host-associated microbes are those in the gastrointestinal tract. In the area of infectious diseases and infection control, we typically look at individual diseases caused by single organisms. Conventionally microbes are thought of as bad actors because the emphasis is on disease rather than interaction between human and microbial cells. The protective role of a large number of bacterial species that exist on and around us has largely been minimized. In fact, these bacteria should be referred to as "Nature's Bioshield." Their association with the areas they were put in by nature is strong and symbiotic. Since they are common to healthy individuals, their transmission from person to person is of no relevance. We know now that the disruption of this bioshield by physical injury and its alteration by the selection process from antibiotic use are the most significant risk factors for developing infectious diseases including those caused by multiple antibiotic-resistant bacteria and their transmission to others in the health-care as well as community settings.

The transmission from person to person was proven even before the germ theory of disease was proven. For example, in 1841, Ignaz Semmelweis, a Hungarian physician, attempted to mandate hand washing and change of coats used in autopsy rooms before examining patients or performing deliveries. He believed that invisible agents can be transferred particularly from autopsy room to delivery room thus infecting mothers during birthing. He built this belief from his observation that the death rates in the ward that was run by physicians were 18 % more than that in the ward run by midwives. He contributed that to the fact that physicians were working in autopsy rooms and the midwives were not. Also one of his colleagues died after he cut himself during an autopsy on a patient who had died from puerperal fever/sepsis. His colleagues did not accept the concept despite the fact that the death rate in the hospital dropped by 66 % after applying the two interventions. It is difficult to comprehend why Dr. Semmelweis faced opposition despite the success of his measures. The question was and remains today: Is it hard to apply these practices or are we not able to meaningfully convey the principles?

Historically, the concept of cleaning and sanitizing was practiced long before the germ theory was conceived, it is all about cleaning. Even the theories developed in the middle ages about cleaning said that diseases were caused by the presence of "miasma" in the air. Miasma is a poisonous vapor with a foul smell. This theory encouraged people to get rid of the foul smell by cleaning which helped decrease the rate of diseases by getting rid of what later was named as germs.

It was the effort of many scientists to develop and prove the germ theory. The first step was taken by Antoni Van Leeuwenhoek who saw tiny structures under the microscope in 1677 and called them "animalcules."

The germ theory of disease was well established in the early 1880s based on Robert Koch's published work on tubercle bacillus. In 1882, one of his assistants Friedrich Loeffler published the three postulates that need to be fulfilled to establish an association between a microbe and a disease process (Box 1.1). These postulates were formalized by Koch himself between 1884 and 1890. Concurrent with establishing the pathogenicity of the limited number of bacteria, the transmission pathways and their interruption

Box 1.1

Loeffler's postulate	Koch's postulate
1. The organisms must be shown to be constantly present in characteristic form and arrangement in the disease tissue	1. The same organism must be present in every case of the disease
2. The organisms, which from their behavior appear to be responsible for the disease, must be isolated and cultivated in purity	2. The organism must be isolated from the diseased host and grown in pure culture
3. The pure cultures must be shown to include disease experimentally	3. The isolate must cause the disease, when inoculated into a healthy, susceptible animal
	4. The organism must be reisolated from the inoculated, diseased animal

were being conceived also. Joseph Lister and John Snow contributed significantly to the acceptance of germ theory.

A century and quarter later, everybody seems to agree with the importance of prevention and its application but the compliance is still an issue. Perhaps this is because the consequences of noncompliance are not obvious right away and it is hard to point to a single action that caused the incident. It is a fact that those we ask to comply with infection prevention practices do not have a clear understanding of the microbial world at large and therefore the principles. This has made it difficult and at times impossible to have an optimal adherence with these practices. We believe that it is absolutely necessary to convey to health-care providers of all levels the significance of the microbial flora on and around us, the factors that put them at risk for acquiring and subsequently transmitting disease-causing pathogens to patients at high risk of developing infectious processes due to multiple factors including age, immunocompromise, and comorbid conditions. With that in mind the rest of this chapter will provide an overview of bacteria, viruses, prions, fungi, and parasites with focus on modes of transmission and therefore the modes of prevention of transmission. The details of the procedures to reduce transmission in the health-care settings will be provided in the following chapters.

Pathogenic Bacteria and Their Modes of Transmission

Bacteria by definition lack membrane-enclosed nucleus and membrane-enclosed organelles like mitochondria and chloroplast. They have double-stranded DNA and a cell wall made of peptido-glycan. Based on the amount of the peptidoglycan in the cell wall, bacteria will retain crystal violet during the gram-staining process and not get decolorized which gives them a purple color and therefore are classified as gram-positive bacteria.

In contrast, gram-negative bacteria have a thin layer of peptidoglycan, are decolorized after the initial staining by crystal violet, and take the counter stain safranin. These bacteria acquire pink in color and are classified as gram negative. The bacteria of clinical relevance are further classified based on their morphology that is spherical or cocci or rod shaped or bacilli. The cocci can be present in clusters such as staphylo-cocci or in chains such as streptococci. The third level of classification is based on the growth under aerobic and anaerobic conditions. Most aerobic bacteria are able to also grow under anaerobic condition and are facultative anaer-obes. Obligate anaerobes, on the other hand, grow only in the absence of oxygen. Further identification to the genus and the species level is determined by biochemical reactions (pheno-typic characteristics) and/or molecular tech-niques (genotypic characteristics).

Gram-Positive Bacteria

Gram-positive aerobic cocci	Gram-positive anaerobic cocci	Gram-positive aerobic bacilli	Gram-positive anaerobic bacilli
Staphylococcus	Peptostreptococcus	Bacillus	Clostridium
Streptococcus	Peptococcus	Corynebacterium	Actinomycete
Enterococcus		Listeria	
		Nocardia	

Aerobic Gram-Positive Cocci

Staphylococci are aerobic/facultatively anaerobic gram-positive cocci that are not motile and do not form spores. Of the 31 species recognized, Staphylococcus aureus and Staphylococcus intermedius produce the enzyme coagulase which helps in their identification and is also a virulence factor.

S. aureus colonizes the skin and mucous membranes of 30–50 % of healthy adults and children, most commonly in the anterior nares, skin, vagina, and rectum [1]. In addition to coag-ulase, S. aureus has a number of virulence factors including exotoxins such as enterotoxin, exfolia-tive toxin, and toxic shock syndrome toxin 1. The primary sites of infections caused by S. aureus

are the skin and soft tissue; however, infection can become disseminated, causing bloodstream infection and multiple organ involvement includ-ing endocarditis. The point of entry of S. aureus maybe obvious such as folliculitis or maybe related to skin disruption which is not obvious. In addition, S. aureus can colonize devices following transcutaneous insertion producing a biofilm on the device with subsequent potential for bloodstream infection and dissemination. The ingestion of food contaminated with S. aureus can cause food poisoning due to the presence of preformed enterotoxin.

Transmission of S. aureus occurs primarily by contact with the skin of colonized people and/or environmental surfaces which have been contaminated by colonized people. Colonized personnel in the health-care setting serve as reservoir for *S. aureus* transmission to patients and to the surfaces. However, transmission is common even in the community setting. The best example is the recent significant increase in the community-associated skin and soft tissue infections caused by *S. aureus* clone 300. Food contaminated by dietary personnel has been implicated in staphylococcal food poisoning. Transmission of *S. aureus* can be reduced by hand hygiene and decontamination of environmental surfaces.

Coagulase-negative staphylococci (CNS) are present on the skin of all humans and are the most abundant constituent of the normal flora at this site [2]. If and when CNS enter the bloodstream, e.g., through insertion of medical devices, they can cause bloodstream infection, endocarditis in patients with prosthetic valves, infections of pacemakers and intravascular catheters, and other foreign bodies in place. *Staphylococcus* epidermidis accounts for about half of resident staphylococci and majority of the isolates in clinical blood specimens [3]. Other clinically significant species include *S. saprophyticus*, which causes urinary tract infection in young sexually active women, and *S. lugdunensis* which cause endocarditis, osteomyelitis, and septicemia. *S. hominis*, *S. haemolyticus*, *S. warneri,* and *S. simulans* are rarely isolated as pathogens. The most optimal way to prevent infections by CNS is hand hygiene, effective skin antisepsis, and barrier precautions during procedures outside the operating room.

Streptococci are facultatively anaerobic gram-positive cocci that form pairs or chains. Different species cause different infections, so it is important to know the classification. The classification does not depend on a single factor but rather it depends on different factors including hemolytic reaction on blood agar, serologic specificity of cell wall (Lancefield classification), and biochemical characteristics.

The serological classification (Lancefield classification) depends on the carbohydrate antigen in the cell wall based on which streptococci are classified into (A, B, C, etc.).

S. pyogenes, group A (GAS), β-hemolytic, is a common cause of pharyngitis and impetigo. *S. pyogenes* contains cell wall M protein which is an important virulent factor and induces cross-reactive antibodies leading to nonsuppurative complications of rheumatic fever and glomerulonephritis. It can occasionally colonize the respiratory tract and the skin. It can be transmitted from person to person through respiratory droplets to cause pharyngitis or through a break of the skin after direct contact to an infected person, fomite, or arthropod vector to cause skin infection. Nosocomial transmission of GAS to or by personnel can be prevented by hand hygiene and other practices including standard precautions that should be used for every patient contact. Other transmission-based precautions may be needed under special circumstances and outbreak situations.

S. agalactiae, group B (GAS), β-hemolytic, can cause urinary tract infection, postpartum endometritis, and bacteremia in pregnant women and sepsis and meningitis in neonates. Recently it has been recognized as an important cause of sepsis in nonpregnant adults especially those with diabetes mellitus [4]. It can be a part of the flora of the upper respiratory tract and genitourinary tract. The transmission of GBS from the mother's vaginal flora to the newborn during delivery is clearly understood. This has lead to the practice of surveillance cultures for GBS in vaginal flora during antenatal care. There are clear guidelines to manage GBS colonization in pregnant women prior to and during delivery in order to prevent its transmission to the newborn.

Group C and group G (*S. dysgalactiae*) are β-hemolytic streptococci that can cause pharyngitis and cellulitis clinically indistinguishable from GAS disease although they are more commonly opportunistic and nosocomial pathogens. These similarities can be explained by the sharing of a number of virulence factors with GAS like streptolysin and antigens similar to M protein. They can be part of the normal human flora and the transmission is similar to that for GAS.

Viridans streptococci like *S. mitis*, *S. sanguis,* and *S. salivarius* are α-hemolytic and are members of the upper respiratory tract flora and can cause transient bacteremia which makes them the principal cause of endocarditis on abnormal heart valves. *S. mutans* produces polysaccharide that contributes to the genesis of dental caries.

S. pneumoniae is α- or nonhemolytic which can cause pneumonia, meningitis, endocarditis, and disseminated infection. These bacteria are ubiquitous. Most infections are caused by spread from colonized nasopharynx or oropharynx to distal sites (lung, blood, meninges). Person-to-person spread through respiratory droplets is rare.

S. bovis (formerly called nonenterococcal group D streptococci) are nonhemolytic and can cause endocarditis and are commonly isolated in blood in patients with colon cancer. It can colonize the lower gastrointestinal tract and rarely the upper gastrointestinal tract.

Enterococci (formerly called group D streptococci) are gram-positive cocci of intestinal origin that usually form short chains. They are a part of the gastrointestinal flora which is the commonest source of infections caused by enterococci. Rarely person-to-person spread can occur. The infections caused by enterococci include endocarditis, urinary tract infection, wound infection, biliary tract infection, and bacteremia. *E. faecalis* in the most common species and causes 85–90 % of enterococcal infections, while *E. faecium* causes 5–10 %. Some of enterococci, especially *E. faecium*, are vancomycin resistant. In the United States, 80 % of *E. faecium* and 6.9 % of *E. faecalis* were resistant to vancomycin between 2006 and 2007 [5]. Vancomycin-resistant enterococci (VRE) are often multidrug-resistant bacteria, and contact precaution is applied in the hospital settings for prevention of transmission.

Anaerobic Gram-Positive Cocci

Peptococci are obligate anaerobic gram-positive cocci. These bacteria are part of the flora of the mouth, upper respiratory tract, and large intestine. They can cause soft tissue infection and bacteremia.

Peptostreptococci are obligate anaerobic gram-positive cocci that is α- or nonhemolytic. These bacteria are part of the normal flora on the skin and mucous membranes. They can cause abscesses mostly in association with other bacteria.

Aerobic Gram-Positive Bacilli

Bacillus species are aerobic spore-forming gram-positive rods occurring in chains. They are saprophytic organisms prevalent in soil, water, and air. The principle pathogens of this genus are *B. anthracis* and *B. cereus*. *B. anthracis* causes anthrax which occurs when the spores are introduced cutaneously or through inhalation. The inhalation form is more serious but both forms can be complicated by systemic disease and meningitis. In 2001, 22 cases occurred due to bioterrorist attacks through contaminated envelopes which brought awareness to this old pathogen since it was rarely seen in the United states from 1980 to 2000 [6]. *B. cereus* is known to cause food poisoning and occasionally can cause bacteremia. This is a challenging diagnosis as *Bacillus* species are common contaminants in blood cultures and only 5–10 % present bloodstream infection [7].

Corynebacterium: *C. diphtheria* is the most important member of the group and can cause respiratory and cutaneous disease. Asymptomatic carriers accounts for 5 % of the population and are important for the transmission of the disease [8]. It secretes a toxin that inhibits protein synthesis and has necrotizing and neurotoxic effect. Treatment of the carriers and isolation of infected patients are important measures for the prevention of transmission, but the toxoid-based vaccination is the key to the decrease in the incidence of diphtheria.

Listeria species are facultative, motile, nonspore-forming gram-positive rods. *L. monocytogenes* is the most common and can cause a wide spectrum of diseases. It enters through gastrointestinal tract and can cause food-borne infections (1 % of cases of food-borne infections [9]). It can cause septicemia, meningitis, or encephalitis especially in immunocompromised, pregnant women, elderly, and neonates.

Nocardia asteroides complex is the species that is responsible for the majority of the cases of nocardiosis. They are aerobic gram-positive rods but they are also weak acid-fast. Nocardia are found in soil and water and are not transmitted from person to person. Nocardiosis is an opportunistic infection associated with impaired cellular immunity. It causes chronic pneumonia which can mimic tuberculosis and can spread from lung to brain and form abscesses. Disseminated form can spread to skin, kidney, bone, and other systems.

Anaerobic Gram-Positive Bacilli

Clostridium species are anaerobic spore-forming large gram-positive rods which are also saprophytic organisms found in the soil and the intestinal tract of animals and humans. Among the pathogens is *C. botulinum* that causes food poisoning mostly from the canned foods that leads to flaccid paralysis due to the blocking effect of the toxin on the acetylcholine release in the synapse of the neuromuscular junctions. *C. tetani* causes tetanus which is a tonic contraction of the muscles as the toxin blocks the release of the inhibitory mediators like gamma-aminobutyric acid. Both pathogens act through their toxins and are associated with high mortality. *C. botulinum* spores are highly resistant to heat and 20 min of boiling is needed to destroy these spores. For tetanus, the toxoid-based vaccination is the key for prevention.

C. perfringens can cause myonecrosis and gas gangrene when introduced into damaged tissue. The effect is through alpha and theta toxins which can cause rapid and significant damage to the muscles and soft tissues which can rapidly progress to shock and death. In the other hand, ingesting secreted enterotoxin can cause self-limited diarrhea.

C. difficile causes pseudomembranous colitis in patients with exposure to antibiotics. It secretes toxin A and toxin B which are responsible for the disease. Hand washing with soap and water is the only effective way to prevent transmission from patient to patient in the hospital setting. Alcohol-based hand hygiene products do not kill *C. difficile* spores.

Actinomyces are non-spore-forming branching anaerobic filamentous gram-positive bacilli that readily fragment into bacillary forms. They reproduce by binary fission, a feature that differentiates them from fungi [10]. Most are saprophytes and live in soil, but members of this group are responsible for actinomycosis.

Actinomyces israelii is responsible for most of the cases of actinomycosis. It is a part of the human oral flora. It causes chronic disease characterized by abscess formation, draining sinus tracts, fistulae, and tissue fibrosis. Cervicofacial form accounts for half of the cases and also can manifest as central nervous system, thoracic, abdominal, and pelvic infections [11].

Gram-Negative Bacteria

Gram-negative aerobic cocci	Gram-negative anaerobic cocci	Gram-negative aerobic bacilli	Gram-negative anaerobic bacilli
Neisseria	*Veillonella*	*Enterobacteriaceae*	*Bacteroides*
Moraxella		*Pseudomonas*	
		Haemophilus	
		Brucella	
		Bordetella	
		Legionella	
		Chlamydia	
		Mycoplasma	
		Rickettsia	

Aerobic Gram-Negative Cocci

Neisseria are aerobic or facultatively anaerobic gram-negative diplococci. *N. meningitidis* and *N. gonorrhoeae* are pathogenic for humans which are the only host and typically are found associated with or inside polymorphonuclear cells. Other *Neisseria* species are normal inhabitants of the upper respiratory tract; they are extracellular and rarely cause disease.

N. meningitidis can be subdivided into serogroups based on distinct capsular polysaccharides. Eight serogroups most commonly cause infections in humans (A, B, C, X, Y, Z, W135, and L). The organism is considered a respiratory pathogen and spread by the aerosol route. It is clear that the high attack rates seen in the less developed countries are in part due to poverty and a consequence of crowding, poor sanitation, and malnutrition. Infection can produce a variety of clinical manifestations, ranging from transient fever and bacteremia to meningitis and fulminant disease with death ensuing within hours of the onset of clinical symptoms.

CDC recommends two doses of MCV4 (the vaccine that covers serotypes A,C,Y, and W135) for adolescents aging from 11 to 18 years, the first dose at 11 years of age with a booster dose at age 16.

For chemoprophylaxis, CDC recommends for adults or children who within 7 days prior to the onset of meningococcal disease lived or slept in the same household as the patient, have been contacts in the day care center, or directly exposed to the patient's oral secretions (e.g., through kissing, mouth-to-mouth resuscitation, endotracheal intubation, or endotracheal tube management).

For health-care settings, patients infected with *N. meningitidis* are rendered noninfectious by 24 h of effective therapy. Personnel who care for patients with suspected *N. meningitidis* infection can decrease their risk of infection by adhering to droplet precautions. Postexposure prophylaxis is advised for persons who have had intensive, unprotected contact (i.e., without wearing a mask) with infected patients, e.g., mouth-to-mouth resuscitation, endotracheal intubation, endotracheal tube management, or close examination of the oropharynx of patients.

Moraxella catarrhalis is an aerobic gram-negative diplococcus that is an exclusive human pathogen involving the upper respiratory tract. Most children have upper respiratory tract colonization at some point in the first several years of life. Colonization is uncommon in healthy adults, occurring in approximately 1–5 % of individuals [12]. It is a common cause of otitis media in children and acute exacerbations in adults with chronic obstructive pulmonary disease.

Anaerobic Gram-Negative Cocci

Veillonella are small anaerobic gram-negative cocci. They are part of the normal flora of the mouth, nasopharynx, and the intestine. Though occasionally isolated in polymicrobial anaerobic infections, they are rarely the sole cause of infection.

Aerobic Gram-Negative Bacilli

Enterobacteriaceae are aerobic (facultative anaerobic) non-spore-forming gram-negative bacilli. Some enteric organisms like *Escherichia coli* are part of the normal flora and incidentally cause disease, while others like Salmonellae and Shigellae are enteric pathogens for humans.

E. coli, *Proteus*, *Enterobacter*, *Klebsiella*, *Morganella*, *Providencia*, *Citrobacter*, and *Serratia* are members of the normal intestinal flora and can be a part of the normal flora of the upper respiratory and genital tracts. They can be recovered from the gastrointestinal tract of cattle and other mammals, soil, sewage, aquatic environment, contaminated food, water, and medical environment. They can be transient residents on the hands of health-care workers. They are transmitted by "food, fingers, feces, and flies" from person to person, and health-care workers play a significant role in the hospital setting.

They can cause hospital- and community-acquired infections, and some of them like Serratia and Enterobacter are considered opportunistic pathogens. They cause urinary tract infection, pneumonia, bacteremia, wound infections, and meningitis. Some E. coli strains can cause diarrheal diseases, e.g., enterotoxigenic *E. coli* that causes traveler's diarrhea due to exotoxins and enterotoxins and enterohemorrhagic *E. coli* that causes hemorrhagic diarrhea due to the shiga-like toxin, among which the serotype O157:H7 can be associated with hemorrhagic uremic syndrome.

Association for Professionals in Infection Control and Epidemiology (APIC) recommends hand washing, alcohol-based hand hygiene, barrier protection, proper maintenance of equipment, and education as measures to prevent transmission.

CDC recommends personal hygiene including hand washing, cooking meat thoroughly, avoiding consuming raw milk and unpasteurized dairy products, and avoiding swallowing water during swimming.

In case of multiresistant bacteria contact, isolation should be performed to prevent transmission from one patient to another by applying hand hygiene and using gloves and gowns.

Shigellae are limited to the intestinal tract of humans and other primates. Infections are almost always limited to the gastrointestinal tract. The infective dose is low at 10–100 organisms, whereas it usually is 10^5–10^8 for Salmonella and Vibrio [13]. They are also transmitted by "food, fingers, feces, and flies" from person to person. Infections occurred most frequently among children in daycare centers.

Shigella causes diarrhea that is most of the times self-limited, and on recovery most persons shed the bacteria for a short period but few remain chronic intestinal carriers. *S. sonnei* commonly causes mild disease which may be limited to watery diarrhea, while *S. dysenteriae* or *S. flexneri* causes dysenteric symptoms (bloody diarrhea) [14].

CDC recommends hand washing after going to the bathroom, after changing diapers, and before preparing foods or beverages and supervising hand washing of toddlers and small children after they use the toilet. Keeping children with diarrhea out of child care settings and not to prepare food for others while ill with diarrhea are also recommended.

It is important to report the cases of shigellosis to the public health department. If many cases occur at the same time, it may mean that a restaurant or food or water supply has a problem that needs correction by the public health department.

Salmonella: Although there are many types of Salmonella, they can be divided into two broad categories: those that cause typhoid and enteric fever and those that primarily cause gastroenteritis. The typhoidal Salmonella, such as *S. typhi* and *S. paratyphi*, have a high host specificity for humans. Infection virtually always implies contact with an acutely infected individual, a chronic carrier, or contaminated food and water. In the United States, typhoid fever has become less prevalent and is now primarily a disease of travelers and immigrants. The much broader group of nontyphoidal Salmonella is a common cause of food-borne gastroenteritis worldwide, particularly in outbreak settings. Traditionally infection has been associated with raw meat or poultry products and improperly handled food that has been contaminated by animal or human fecal material or via the fecal-oral route, from other humans or farm or pet animals [15].

Enteric (typhoid) fever can be complicated with intestinal bleeding and perforation due to the ileocecal lymphatic hyperplasia. It is usually manifested by fever, bradycardia, abdominal pain, and faint rash. Symptoms gradually resolve over weeks to month.

CDC, besides hand hygiene, recommends that people should avoid eating raw or undercooked eggs, poultry, or meat. People who have salmonellosis should not prepare food for others until their diarrhea has resolved. Many health departments require that restaurant workers with *Salmonella* infection have a stool test showing that they are no longer carrying the *Salmonella* bacterium before they return to work. Reptiles and birds (especially baby chicks) are particularly likely to have *Salmonella*, and it can contaminate their skin. Everyone should immediately wash their hands after touching them, and they are not appropriate pets for small children and should not be in a house that has an infant.

Pseudomonas aeruginosa is a gram-negative aerobic bacillus. The organism is common in the environment, especially in water, even contaminating distilled water [16]. It is also the cause of infections associated with hot tubs and contaminated contact lens solutions. Considerable attention is paid to *P. aeruginosa* as a potential pathogen in hospitals because reservoirs for infection can develop, especially in intensive care units. The organism is an opportunistic pathogen for immunocompromised hosts.

Historically, *P. aeruginosa* has been a major burn wound pathogen, an agent of bacteremia in neutropenic patients and the most important pathogen in cystic fibrosis patients. It can infect many organs; it is the second most common cause of nosocomial pneumonia (17 %), the third most common cause of urinary tract infection (7 %), the fourth most common cause of surgical site infection (8 %), the seventh most frequently isolated pathogen from the bloodstream (2 %), and the fifth most common isolate (9 %) overall from all sites [17].

CDC recommends contact precaution in addition to standard precaution if the organ is resistant to multiple antibiotic classes.

Multidrug-resistant **Pseudomonas aeruginosa** and **Acinetobacter baumannii** are becoming increasingly important nosocomial pathogens worldwide. To study the evolution of non-fermenters in a tertiary care hospital, a 10-year (1999–2008) retrospective trend analysis of antimicrobial consumption and resistance in non-fermenters causing bacteremia was undertaken. A significant increase in resistance in *A. baumannii* to fluoroquinolones ($r^2=0.63$, $P=0.006$), aminoglycosides ($r^2=0.63$, $P=0.011$), and carbapenems ($r^2=0.82$, $P=0.013$) and in *P. aeruginosa* to aminoglycosides ($r^2=0.59$, $P=0.01$) was observed. Carbapenem consumption was associated with the development of resistance in *A. baumannii* ($r=0.756$, $P=0.049$), whereas no such association was observed for other antimicrobials among non-fermenters [18].

Haemophilus is a facultative anaerobic pleomorphic gram-negative rod occurring in pairs or short chains. *H. influenzae type b* is an important human pathogen. *H. ducreyi*, a sexually transmitted pathogen, causes chancroid. Other species are among normal flora of mucous membranes and only occasionally cause disease. Humans are the only known reservoir.

H. influenzae is transmitted by respiratory droplet spread. It has encapsulated (serotypes a through f) and non-encapsulated forms (nontypeable). The most important serotype is *H. influenzae* serotype b (Hib), which was a frequent cause of bacteremia, meningitis, and other invasive infections prior to the routine use of Hib conjugate vaccines in children. Other capsular serotypes and unencapsulated *H. influenzae* strains can also cause disease, mainly mucosal infections (sinusitis, otitis, bronchitis) but occasionally cause more invasive infections.

Hib vaccine induces antibodies to the type b capsular polysaccharide; it is highly protective and is recommended by CDC for all children younger than 5 years old. It is usually given to infants starting at 2 months old.

Chemoprophylaxis is recommended for household contacts defined as persons residing with the index patient or nonresidents who cumulatively spent 4 or more hours with the index case for at least 5 of the 7 days prior to the day of hospital admission and there is a member of the contact's household who is younger than 4 years of age and is unimmunized or incompletely immunized or is an immunocompromised child, regardless of the child's immunization status.

Brucella are small, gram-negative, nonmotile, facultative, intracellular aerobic rods. Brucellosis is a zoonotic infection transmitted to humans by contact with fluids from infected animals (sheep, cattle, goats, pigs, or other animals) or through food products such as unpasteurized milk and cheese. It is one of the most widespread zoonosis worldwide [19]. Clinical manifestations of brucellosis include fever, night sweats, malaise, anorexia, arthralgias, fatigue, weight loss, and depression. It can become chronic and is characterized by localized infections like spondylitis, osteomyelitis, tissue abscesses, and uveitis.

Bordetella pertussis causes pertussis, also known as "whooping cough" which is a highly contagious, acute respiratory illness. In the pre-vaccine era, the disease predominantly affected children less than 10 years of age and usually manifested as a prolonged cough illness with one or more of the classical symptoms, including inspiratory whoop, paroxysmal cough, and post-tussive emesis [20]. Since the introduction of pertussis vaccines, the epidemiology of reported pertussis infections has changed; in the United States in the 1990s, more than one-half of cases occurred in adolescents and adults [21]. Routine childhood vaccination in the United States is performed with the DTaP vaccine (acellular pertussis vaccine combined with tetanus and diphtheria toxoids) and the vaccine efficacy is 92 % [22]. Postexposure antibiotic prophylaxis is warranted for individuals with close contact to a person with pertussis. A close contact is defined as a person who has had face-to-face exposure within 3 ft of a symptomatic patient. Individuals with direct contact with respiratory, nasal, or oral secretions may also be considered close contacts.

Legionellas are aerobic, gram-negative bacilli. *L. pneumophila* is the most common species, which causes at least 80 % of human infections. It can cause community-acquired and hospital-acquired pneumonia. Legionellosis refers to the two clinical syndromes, Legionnaires' disease which is the more common syndrome of pneumonia caused by *Legionella* species and Pontiac fever which is an acute, febrile, self-limited illness with minimal if nay respiratory symptoms. Transmission in facilities has been linked to potable water distribution systems. CDC recommends culturing of the water at sites the patient was exposed to in case of nosocomial legionnaire's disease.

Chlamydias are gram-negative or variable obligate intracellular bacteria. The species that most commonly affect humans are *C. trachomatis*, *C. pneumoniae*, and *C psittaci*. *C. trachomatis* causes sexually transmitted disease that is often asymptomatic but can cause cervicitis in women and urethritis in men. The most serious complication in women is pelvic inflammatory disease that can occur in asymptomatic patients also and can lead to infertility. *C. pneumoniae* and *C. psittaci* cause pneumonia and the transmission of the organism is thought to be person to person.

Mycoplasma pneumoniae is a facultative anaerobic rod that is not visible on gram staining due to the absence of cell wall. It is transmitted from person to person by respiratory droplets during close contact [23]. Patients with respiratory infection caused by *M. pneumoniae* may have cough, pharyngitis, rhinorrhea, and ear pain; only 10 % of patients develop pneumonia. Extrapulmonary manifestations are hemolysis, skin rash, and rarely central nervous system complications.

Rickettsia: Rocky Mountain spotted fever (RMSF) is a potentially lethal but usually curable tick-borne disease. The etiologic agent, *Rickettsia rickettsii*, is a gram-negative, obligate intracellular bacterium. The clinical spectrum of human infection with *R. rickettsii* ranges from mild to fulminant. In the early phases of illness, most patients have nonspecific signs and symptoms such as fever, headache, malaise, myalgias, and nausea. Rash appears between the third and fifth days of illness. RMSF occurs throughout the United States, in Canada, Mexico, Central America, and in parts of South America. In the United States, it is most prevalent in the southeastern and south central states. RMSF is usually transmitted via a tick bite. Tick bites are painless and up to one-third of patients with proven RMSF do not recall a recent tick bite.

Scrub typhus is a rickettsial disease caused by the organism *Orientia tsutsugamushi* and is transmitted to humans by the bite of a larval-stage trombiculid mite or chigger. Scrub typhus is widespread in the so-called tsutsugamushi triangle which includes Japan, Taiwan, China, and South Korea on the north, India and Nepal on the west, and Australia and Indonesia on the south. Epidemics of scrub typhus have been reported from various parts of the Indian subcontinent [24–27].

It presents as either a nonspecific febrile illness with constitutional symptoms such as fever, rash, myalgias, and headache or with organ dysfunctions involving organs such as kidney (acute renal failure, ARF), liver (hepatitis), lungs (acute respiratory distress syndrome, ARDS), central nervous system (meningitis), or with circulatory collapse with hemorrhagic features. Scrub typhus is one of the differential diagnoses (in addition to leptospirosis, malaria, or dengue fever) in patients with hemorrhagic fever especially if associated with jaundice and/or renal failure.

Anaerobic Gram-Negative Bacilli

Bacteroides are anaerobic gram-negative bacilli and are normal inhabitants of the bowel. They can cause intra-abdominal abscess and peritonitis after bowel injury, most of the times in association with other bacteria.

Spirochetes

Treponema pallidum organisms are slender spirals that are actively motile as seen on dark field microscopy. It causes syphilis which is a chronic infection. The initial clinical manifestations of primary syphilis consist of a painless chancre at the site of inoculation, which usually heals within a few weeks. Few months later, approximately 25 % of individuals with untreated primary infection develop secondary syphilis characterized by systemic symptoms including fever, rash, headache, malaise, anorexia, and diffuse lymphadenopathy. Asymptomatic patients who have *Treponema pallidum* infection by serologic testing alone have "latent syphilis." Patients in the early latent period (within 1 year of primary infection) are believed to be potentially infectious in contrast to late latency when transmission is no longer likely. When patients are untreated during the earlier stages of syphilis, they are at risk for major complications involving the central nervous system or cardiovascular structures or granulomatous disease of the skin or bones. Syphilis is sexually transmitted, except for cases resulting from vertical transmission (i.e., infection acquired in utero or during delivery). Syphilis is transmissible during early disease (primary and secondary syphilis) and early latent disease.

Borrelia burgdorferi causes Lyme disease which is a tick-borne illness. It is responsible of all cases in the United States. In Europe, *B. afzelii* and *B. garinii* are additional responsible species. Borrelia is a spirochete; it is motile, spiral, and cannot be seen by standard light microscopy because of its small size. Lyme disease has three phases; early localized disease manifests as erythema migrans (EM) and nonspecific findings that resemble a viral syndrome, usually occurring within 1 month of the tick bite. Early disseminated disease manifests as acute neurologic or cardiac involvement, usually occurring several weeks to several months after the tick bite. Late disseminated disease manifests as arthritis and neurological manifestations, and in Europe skin manifestations occur months to a few years after the onset of infection. It is transmitted by small ticks called Ixodes. Deer and mice constitute the main animal reservoir. It is endemic in the northeastern and Midwestern parts of the United States, parts of Asia, and parts of Europe.

Leptospira are spiral-shaped aerobic spirochetes; they tend to stain poorly with common laboratory stains and are best visualized by dark field microscopy. The majority of leptospirosis cases occur in the tropics, although cases are also observed in temperate regions. The natural hosts for the organism are various mammals; man is only incidentally infected. The disease leptospirosis (Weil's disease) is associated with a variable clinical course. The disease may manifest as a subclinical illness followed by seroconversion, a self-limited systemic infection, or a severe, potentially fatal illness accompanied by multiorgan failure. Humans most often become infected after exposure to environmental sources, such as animal urine, contaminated water, or soil or infected animal tissue through cuts or abraded skin, mucous membranes, or conjunctiva. Vaccination of domestic animals against leptospirosis provides substantial protection. The major control measure available for humans is to avoid potential sources of infection such as stagnant water, rodent control, and protection of food from animal contamination. No vaccine is available for humans.

Mycobacteria

Mycobacteria are rod-shaped, aerobic bacteria that do not stain readily but when stained they resist decolorization by alcohol or acid leading to the popular reference of acid-fast bacteria. *M. tuberculosis* causes tuberculosis, *M. leprae* causes leprosy, and *M. avium complex* and other atypical mycobacteria are opportunistic infections that occasionally cause disease in immunocompetent patients.

Tuberculosis (TB) is the second most common infectious cause of death in adults worldwide (HIV is the most common). It can affect every organ system. The clinical manifestations are fatigue, weight loss, and fever. Pulmonary involvement causes chronic cough and hemoptysis can be seen in advanced stage. Bloodstream dissemination leads to miliary tuberculosis with lesions in many organs. Latent tuberculosis occurs when the bacteria are present but not manifested by clinical disease and it might become active years later. The people with latent tuberculosis have a 10 % chance to have active tuberculosis in their life, while HIV patients with latent tuberculosis can have active disease more frequently, as high as 5–10 % a year. The human host is the natural reservoir for *M. tuberculosis*. Person-to-person transmission occurs via inhalation of droplet nuclei [28]. Close household contact with an individual with smear-positive pulmonary TB is the most important risk factor for TB. The effective way to prevent tuberculosis is by diagnosing and treating active and latent diseases. Airborne precautions are applied in health-care setting for suspected and confirmed cases of tuberculosis. BCG, a live vaccine for tuberculosis, is an attenuated stain of *M. bovis*. Studies have shown a wide range of effectiveness, from 0 % to 80 %. It is used in endemic area and result in a positive PPD test which wanes with time. The recommendation is to interpret the PPD test without considering the history of BBG vaccine as the chance of having latent tuberculosis with positive PPD is much higher than the chance to have positive test due to BCG vaccine.

Leprosy (Hansen's disease) caused by *M. leprae* involves the skin and peripheral nerves. It is an important global health concern. Early diagnosis and a full course of treatment are critical for preventing lifelong neuropathy and disability. Although the mode of transmission of Hansen's disease remains uncertain, most investigators think that *M. leprae* is usually spread from person to person in respiratory droplets. In the United States, contact with armadillos (handling, killing, or eating) has been reported as a mode of transmission in some cases [29]. BCG vaccine can be used for leprosy in addition to tuberculosis; a single dose appears to be 50 % protective, and two doses further increase protection. Development of an improved BCG vaccine, BCG booster, or alternate vaccine strain is an important research goal that could benefit control of both tuberculosis and leprosy [30].

Pathogenic Viruses and Their Modes of Transmission

Viruses can be transmitted by different modes, the common ones being sexual contact, blood products, respiratory droplets, and direct contact.

Herpes virus family includes herpes simplex virus type 1 (HSV1), herpes simplex virus type 2 (HSV2), varicella-zoster virus, cytomegalovirus, Epstein-Barr virus, and human herpes viruses 6, 7, and 8. Once a patient has become infected by a herpes virus, the infection remains for life. The initial infection may be followed by latency with subsequent reactivation. Each has double-stranded DNA. The viral membrane is quite fragile and a virus with a damaged envelope is not infectious which means that the virus can only be acquired by direct contact with mucosal surfaces or secretions of an infected person.

HSV1 and HSV2: The virus is found in the lesions on the skin and mucous membranes but can also be present in a variety of body fluids including saliva and vaginal secretions. Both types of HSV can infect oral or genital mucosa depending on the regions of contact. HSV1 is usually spread mouth to mouth (kissing or the use of utensils contaminated with saliva) or by transfer of infectious virus to the hands, after which the virus may enter the body via any wound or through the eyes. HSV2 is more commonly spread through sexual contact.

In primary herpetic gingivostomatitis, the typical clear lesions first develop followed by ulcers that have a white appearance. The infection, often initially on the lips spreads to all parts of the mouth and pharynx. Reactivation from the trigeminal ganglia can result in what are known as "cold sores."

Genital herpes is usually caused by HSV2 with about 10 % of cases being the result of HSV1 infection. Primary infection is often asymptomatic but many painful lesions can develop on the glans or shaft of the penis in men and on the vulva, vagina, cervix, and perianal region in women.

Secondary episodes of genital herpes, which occur as a result of reactivation of the virus in the sacral ganglion, are less severe and last a shorter time than the first episode. Recurrent episodes usually follow a primary HSV2 infection. Patients who are about to experience a recurrence usually experience a prodrome in which there is a burning sensation in the area that is about to erupt. Whether there is an active disease or not, an infected patient remains infectious even without overt symptoms. Clearly, these persons are a significant reservoir in the spread of genital herpes virus infection.

Varicella-Zoster virus: This virus causes two major diseases, chicken pox (varicella) usually in childhood and shingles (zoster) later in life. Shingles is a reactivation of an earlier varicella infection.

This virus is highly infectious and more than 90 % of the population of the United States has antibodies against varicella proteins including those with no history of chicken pox. In the household of an infected patient, 90 % of contacts who have not had the disease will get it (unless vaccinated). Spreading of the infection can be from virus in the respiratory tract (by a cough) or from contact with ruptured vesicles on the skin containing infectious virus. Thus, the contagious period can be up to 12–14 days after the initial infection. The disease is more severe in older children and adults. This is particularly the case in immunocompromised patients (AIDS, transplantation, etc.) where the disease may last for several weeks and the fever may be more pronounced. The spread of the virus may lead to infections in the lungs, liver, and in the meninges with mortality up to 20 %.

Shingles: After the infectious period, the virus may migrate to the ganglia where the virus will be dormant. The virus may then be reactivated under stress or with immune suppression. This usually occurs later in life. Lesions occur in restricted areas (dermatomes) that are innervated by a single ganglion. Reactivation can lead to chronic burning or itching pain called post-herpetic neuralgia which is seen primarily in the elderly.

Congenital varicella syndrome is caused by infection in utero during the first trimester. It leads to scarring of the skin of the limbs; damage to the lens, retina, and brain; and microphthalmia.

Epstein-Barr virus is the causative agent of Burkitt's lymphoma in Africa and infectious mononucleosis in the west. The primary infection is often asymptomatic but the patient may shed virus for many years. Some patients develop infectious mononucleosis after 1–2 months of infection. The disease is characterized by malaise, lymphadenopathy, tonsillitis, enlarged spleen and liver, and fever. A large proportion of the population (90–95 %) is infected with Epstein-Barr virus and, although usually asymptomatic, will shed the virus from time to time throughout life. The virus is spread by close contact (kissing disease).

Cytomegalovirus: The virus is spread in most secretions, particularly saliva, urine, vaginal secretions, and semen (which shows the highest titer of any body fluid). *Cytomegalovirus* infection is therefore sexually transmitted. It can also spread to a fetus in a pregnant woman and to the newborn via lactation, though there is some doubt about the importance of milk transmission. In the hospital, the virus can also be spread via blood transfusions and transplants. In third world countries with more crowded conditions, the virus is found in a much higher proportion of the population than in western countries.

During a primary infection of the mother, the virus can spread via the placenta to the fetus and congenital abnormalities can occur. In patients who have received an organ transplant or have an immunosuppressive disease (e.g., AIDS), cytomegalovirus can be a major problem. Particularly important is cytomegalovirus retinitis which occurs in up to 15 % of all AIDS patients. In addition, interstitial pneumonia, colitis, esophagitis, and encephalitis can occur.

Human herpes viruses 6 and 7: These viruses can be isolated from saliva of the majority of adults. They cause exanthem subitum, otherwise known as roseola infantum.

Human herpes virus 8: This was formerly known as Kaposi's sarcoma associated herpes virus and is found in the saliva of many patients with HIV infection/AIDS.

Herpes B virus: This is a simian virus found in old-world monkeys such as macaques, but it can be a human pathogen in people who handle monkeys (monkey bites are the route of transmission). In humans, the disease is much more severe than it is in its natural host. About 75 % of human cases result in death with serious neurological problems (encephalitis) in many survivors. There is some evidence that the disease can be transmitted from a monkey-infected human to another human.

Rubella begins with a prodrome consisting of headache, malaise, fever, and lymphadenopathy followed by the maculopapular rash that lasts for 3 days. The patient is contagious 1 week before and 1–2 weeks after the onset of the rash. Not all patients will have classical symptoms and sometimes symptoms are very mild. The virus can cause congenital rubella if it occurs in the first trimester; it can manifests as fetal death, premature delivery, and congenital rubella syndrome with hearing loss, developmental delay, growth retardation, and cardiac and ophthalmic defects. The virus is shed in respiratory secretions and transmitted through contact or droplet transmission and the humans are the only natural host. Prior to the vaccine, outbreaks of rubella occurred variably every few years. It is rare since the use of routine vaccination (MMR) that is given in two doses at 12–15 months and at 6 years. The rate of immunization is about 100 % in the developed countries but in developing countries still less than 50 % [31].

Measles is characterized by the prodrome phase of fever, malaise, and anorexia followed by conjunctivitis, coryza, cough, and then the rash. The humans are the only host for this virus and the patient is considered contagious 4 days before and 4 days after the rash. Measles can be severe especially in immunocompromised patient and it is the most highly contagious diseases known. The vaccine is very effective and is part of MMR vaccine. Measles virus replicates in the nose, mouth, and throat of the infected person and is dispersed into the air when the ill person coughs, sneezes, or talks. The virus remains viable and contagious for up to 2 h in the air or on surfaces; therefore, transmission can occur without face-to-face contact. Those who are not immune may become infected by inhaling the virus, having contact with droplets containing the virus, or by touching a contaminated surface and then touching the mouth or nose. CDC strategies to prevent nosocomial transmission of measles include documentation of measles immunity in health-care personnel, prompt identification and isolation of persons with fever and rash, and adherence to airborne precautions for suspected and proven cases of measles.

Mumps infection is frequently accompanied by a nonspecific prodrome consisting of low-grade fever, malaise, headache, myalgia, and anorexia followed within 48 h by the development of parotitis. The possible complications of mumps are meningitis, encephalitis, and orchitis. Symptomatic infection in adults is usually more severe than in children. The humans are the only host and the patient is contagious 2 days before and 9 days after the parotitis. The virus is typically transmitted by respiratory droplets or direct contact [32]. Vaccination is effective and is a part of MMR vaccine.

Influenza occurs in outbreaks of varying extent every year. This epidemiologic pattern reflects the changing nature of the antigenic properties of influenza viruses. Influenza begins with the abrupt onset of fever, headache, and myalgia accompanied by manifestations of respiratory tract illness such as nonproductive cough, sore throat, and nasal discharge. The major complication of influenza is pneumonia, which occurs most frequently at the extreme of age and in patients with underlying chronic illnesses. People with Influenza can spread it to others up to 6 ft away. It is spread mainly by droplets directly and indirectly by touching a surface or object that has the virus on it and then touching one's own mouth or nose. There are two main types of flu virus, types A and B. In addition to humans, animals like ducks, chickens, pigs, whales, horses, and seals can also be the host for type A virus, while the humans are the only hosts for type B. Patients are contagious one day before symptoms develop and up to 5–7 days after. In 2010, the Advisory Committee on Immunization Practices (ACIP) for the first time recommended annual influenza vaccination for all persons aged ≥6 months in the United States. Although vaccination is the primary mode of prevention in the community, patients with Influenza should be under droplet precautions while in the hospital.

Although avian influenza A viruses usually do not infect humans, rare cases of human infection with avian influenza A viruses have been reported. Most human infections with avian influenza A viruses have occurred following direct or close contact with infected poultry.

Swine influenza viruses do not normally infect humans. However, sporadic human infections with swine influenza viruses have occurred. Most commonly, human infections with swine viruses occur in people with exposure to infected pigs but there have been documented cases of limited spread of swine influenza viruses from person to person.

Respiratory syncytial virus (RSV) causes seasonal outbreaks of respiratory tract illness throughout the world, usually during the winter season. Almost all children are infected by 2 years of age but it is common among adults also. The infection starts as upper respiratory tract infection with sneezing, rhinorrhea, cough, and sometimes fever and can spread to lower respiratory tract, especially in young children, the elderly, and patients with cardiopulmonary diseases. Direct contact is the most common route of transmission, but large aerosol droplets also have been implicated [3]. Hand washing and contact precautions are used to prevent nosocomial spread. Immunoprophylaxis is available to prevent severe RSV illness in certain infants and children who are at high risk. Researchers are working to develop RSV vaccines, but none is available yet.

Parvovirus (B19): The majority of infected individuals will either be asymptomatic or have nonspecific flu-like symptoms of malaise, muscle pain, and fever. The others will present with the classic symptoms of B19 infection including rash (erythema infectiosum) and arthralgia (fifth disease). It can cause transient aplastic crisis in those with chronic hemolytic disorders and chronic pure red blood cell aplasia in immuno-compromised individuals. The only known host for B19 is humans. The respiratory tract secretions are likely to be an important source of infectious virus and virus gain entry through the respiratory tract. Transmission occurs by large droplets through close contact with the infected person and fomites. The other modes of transmission are vertical transmission during pregnancy and hematogenous transmission through blood products. Infection during pregnancy can result in fetal complications including miscarriage and nonimmune hydrops fetalis. Until a vaccine becomes available, good hygienic practices should be the focus of prevention strategies as it has been shown that hand washing and not sharing food or drinks can at least partially prevent the spread of the virus.

Rhinovirus is one of the most common etiologic agents of the common cold and may play a role in asthma exacerbations. The nasopharynx is the initial site of infection and the virus remains in the nasal secretions for 5–7 days and can be transmitted through small-particle and large-particle aerosol.

Adenovirus: Most adenoviral diseases are self-limited, although fatal infections can occur in immunocompromised hosts and occasionally in healthy children and adults [33]. Most commonly, it causes upper respiratory tract syndromes, but it can also cause pneumonia, gastrointestinal, and ophthalmologic symptoms. Transmission can occur via aerosol droplets, the fecal-oral route, and by contact with contaminated fomites. Adenoviruses can cause significant nosocomial infections. Prolonged infection control measures may be necessary to ensure elimination of adenovirus following a nosocomial outbreak. Oral adenovirus vaccine is approved for use in US military personnel aged 17 through 50 years [34].

Enteroviruses include polioviruses, groups A and B coxsackieviruses, echoviruses, and enteroviruses.

Most of the cases are asymptomatic or result in an undifferentiated febrile illness. Other clinical manifestations of disease include exanthems, enanthems, myopericarditis, and meningitis. Paralytic poliomyelitis which is a known complication of infection due to polioviruses has been eradicated in the United States and other developed countries due to successful vaccination strategies. Poliomyelitis is targeted for worldwide eradication. These viruses are ubiquitous throughout the world and are transmitted from person to person through fecal-oral contact. Simple hygienic measures, such as hand washing, are important to prevent the spread.

Human papillomavirus (HPV): There are more than 100 types of HPV. Some infect skin causing warts (like HPV types 1, 2, and 4), some infect mucous membranes causing genital warts or condyloma acuminatum (like HPV types 6 and 11 that account together for 90 % of genital warts), and some cause intraepithelial neoplasm in the genital area and cervical cancer (like HPV types 16 and 18 that account together for 70 % of all cervical cancer). HPV genotypes can be broadly split into high risk and low risk based upon their association with the development of cervical cancer. HPV only infects humans. Close personal contact is assumed to be of importance for the transmission of cutaneous warts, while anogenital and cervical infection are primarily transmitted through sexual contact. Vaccine plays an important role in prevention. Two vaccines are available. The quadrivalent vaccine (Gardasil) includes HPV types 6, 11, 16, and 18 and prevents genital warts and intraepithelial neoplasia. The bivalent vaccine (Cervarix™) includes HPV types 16 and 18 and prevents intraepithelial neoplasia. Routine immunization should be offered to girls and boys 11–12 years of age but can be administered as early as 9 years. Catch-up vaccination should be offered for females aged 13–26 years and males aged 13–21.

The human immunodeficiency virus (HIV) is a retrovirus, which infects humans when it comes in contact with tissues such as those that line the vagina, anal area, mouth, and eyes or through a break in the skin. Three stages of HIV infection have been described. The initial stage of infection (primary infection), which occurs within weeks of acquiring the virus, is characterized by a flu- or mono-like illness that is seen in about half of the patients and generally resolves within weeks. In this stage there is a rapid increase in plasma viremia, with high viral titers and widespread dissemination targeting lymphoid organs especially the GART. The patients are highly contagious in this stage. This phase is followed by a marked reduction in the virus to steady-state levels probably because of vigorous antivirus cellular responses. The immune response probably accounts for the mono-like or flu-like acute retroviral syndrome. The second stage, a chronic asymptomatic infection lasts an average of 8–10 years. The third stage is the acquired immune deficiency syndrome stage in which the patient is at high risk for opportunistic infections, cancers, severe weight loss, and dementia. The most common modes of infection are sexual transmission at the genital or colonic mucosa, exposure to other infected fluids such as blood or blood products, transmission from mother to infant, and, occasionally, accidental occupational exposure. Due to rapid genetic changes in the virus, there is as yet no vaccine against this infection. Post exposure prophylaxis is used for occupational and nonoccupational exposure and most experts recommend three antiretroviral drugs for 4 weeks.

Hepatitis B: The spectrum of clinical manifestations of hepatitis B virus (HBV) infection varies in both acute and chronic diseases. During the acute phase, manifestations range from subclinical or anicteric hepatitis (70 %) to icteric hepatitis (30 %) and, in some cases, fulminant hepatitis (0.1–0.5 %). During the chronic phase, manifestations range from an asymptomatic carrier state to chronic hepatitis, cirrhosis, and hepatocellular carcinoma. When symptomatic, a patient with acute infection may have anorexia, nausea, jaundice, and right upper quadrant discomfort that lasts from 1 to 3 months, and 5 % of adults will develop chronic disease compared to 90 % if infected at birth [35]. The method of acquiring HBV infection varies geographically. Perinatal transmission is most common in high prevalence areas such as the southeast Asia and China, while sexual contact and percutaneous transmission (e.g., intravenous drug use) are most common in the United States, Canada, and western Europe. Vaccination is highly effective (90 % effectiveness in immunocompetent) and it can be given safely to pregnant women. The Advisory Committee on Immunization Practices (ACIP) recommends that all children receive their first dose of hepatitis B vaccine at birth and complete the vaccine series by age 6–18 months. Older children and adolescents who did not previously receive the hepatitis B vaccine should also be vaccinated. After exposure to hepatitis B virus (HBV), whether it is occupational or nonoccupational, appropriate and timely prophylaxis can prevent HBV infection and subsequent development of chronic infection or liver disease. People who completed hepatitis B vaccine series and did not receive post-vaccination testing should receive a single booster vaccine dose, while unvaccinated persons should receive both hepatitis B immune globulin and hepatitis B vaccine as soon as possible after exposure (preferably within 24 h). The same approach is used for children born to infected mothers. Hepatitis B vaccine may be administered simultaneously with HBIG through a separate injection site.

Hepatitis C: Most acutely infected patients are asymptomatic or have a clinically mild course; jaundice is present in fewer than 25 %. Acute HCV infection typically leads to chronic infection in 60–80 % of cases. Percutaneous transmission (e.g., intravenous drug use) is the most common mode of transmission. Perinatal transmission and sexual contact are also possible modes of transmission. Most scientific evidence demonstrates that although HCV can be transmitted sexually, such transmission happens rarely, so patients with one long-term, steady sex partner do not need to change their sexual practices. However, heterosexual and homosexual persons with concurrent HIV infection or with more than one partner are at risk and should use condoms. Women do not need to avoid pregnancy or breast-feeding, but patients should be advised that approximately six of every 100 infants born to HCV-infected woman become

HCV infected. HCV has not been shown to be transmitted through breast-feeding. Testing to determine whether HCV infection has developed is recommended for health-care workers after percutaneous or per mucosal exposures to HCV-positive blood. Children born to HCV-positive women also should be tested as prompt identification of acute infection is important, because outcomes are improved when treatment is initiated earlier in the course of illness. No postexposure prophylaxis has been demonstrated to be effective against HCV. Immune globulin has no role in prevention and no vaccine for hepatitis C is available.

Rabies viruses: Rabies is virtually always fatal, but disease can be prevented with proper wound care and post exposure prophylaxis. The first symptoms of rabies may be very similar to those of the influenza including general weakness, discomfort, fever, and headache. These symptoms may last for days before progressing to symptoms of cerebral dysfunction, anxiety, confusion, agitation, delirium, hydrophobia, and insomnia. The rabies virus is transmitted through saliva or brain/nervous system tissue.

Transmission of rabies virus usually begins when infected saliva of a host is passed to an uninfected animal. The most common mode of rabies virus transmission is through the bite and virus-containing saliva of an infected host. Transmission has been rarely documented via other routes such as contamination of mucous membranes (i.e., eyes, nose, mouth), aerosol transmission, and corneal and organ transplantations. All species of mammals are susceptible to rabies virus infection but only a few species are important as reservoirs for the disease. In the United States, distinct strains of rabies virus have been identified in raccoons, skunks, foxes, coyotes, and bats which play an important role in transmission. In developing countries dogs are the primary source. Postexposure prophylaxis consists of a regimen of one dose of immune globulin and four doses of rabies vaccine over a 14-day period. Preexposure prophylaxis should be targeted to persons in high-risk groups, including veterinarians, laboratory workers, and international travelers.

Yellow fever virus causes yellow fever which has a high case fatality rate. It starts with nonspecific symptoms and signs including fever, malaise, headache, and joint pains followed by a period of remission lasting up to 48 h followed by a systemic illness which is characterized by hepatic dysfunction, renal failure, coagulopathy, and shock. CDC recommends immunization for travelers to yellow fever endemic areas of Africa and South America and for residents of those areas.

West Nile virus causes West Nile fever characterized by fever, headache, malaise, back pain, anorexia, and a maculopapular rash that appears in approximately one-half of patients. It can present as encephalitis, meningitis, or an acute asymmetric flaccid paralysis. It is found in the Americas, southern Europe, western parts of Asia, Russia, Australia, and Africa. Wild birds serve as hosts but generally remain asymptomatic. No human vaccine is yet available.

St. Louis encephalitis virus: Infection with SLE virus only rarely results in clinical illness but encephalitis can occur especially in elderly patients. The virus is widely distributed in the Americas.

Japanese encephalitis virus: The most common presentation of JEV infection is acute encephalitis but it can manifest as aseptic meningitis or a nonspecific febrile illness with headache. Pigs and wading birds are considered amplifying hosts. Humans are incidental and dead-end hosts for JEV as they do not develop sufficiently high viremia to infect feeding mosquitoes.

Dengue: The clinical manifestations of dengue range from self-limited dengue fever to dengue hemorrhagic fever with shock syndrome which is more common than the self-limited form. Dengue viruses are endemic in every continent except Europe and Antarctica. To date, there is no licensed vaccine available for preventing dengue.

Yellow fever virus, West Nile virus, St. Louis encephalitis virus, Japanese encephalitis viruses, and dengue virus are members of the family Flaviviridae and are transmitted by mosquito. Personal protection measures include the use of mosquito repellents and mosquito nets.

Prions and Their Mode of Transmission

Prions are small infectious pathogens containing protein but lack nucleic acid. Prion diseases are neurodegenerative diseases that have long incubation periods and progress rapidly once clinical symptoms appear. Five human prion diseases are currently recognized: kuru, Creutzfeldt-Jakob disease (CJD), variant Creutzfeldt-Jakob disease (vCJD), Gerstmann-Sträussler-Scheinker syndrome (GSS), and fatal familial insomnia (FFI). Bovine spongiform encephalopathy (BSE), one of a number of prion infections affecting animals, was responsible for bringing these agents to more widespread public attention because of its link to vCJD. Prion diseases appear to result from neurotoxic accumulation of abnormal isoforms of the prion protein. The gene encoding the prion protein in humans is located on the short arm of chromosome 20. A strong link was established between mutations in this gene and forms of prion disease with a familial predisposition (familial Creutzfeldt-Jakob disease, Gerstmann-Sträussler-Scheinker syndrome, and fatal familial insomnia). The two diseases that are thought to be due to transmission of prions are kuru and vCJD. In kuru, symptoms begin with tremors, ataxia, and postural instability followed by loss of ambulation and involuntary movements. Dementia progresses in the late stages of the disease, with death typically occurring within 9–24 months from the onset. It is felt to be transmitted from person to person. Cannibalism which was common in New Guinea in the past could be the reason why it was endemic there. Now as this practice has been stopped, kuru has become rare. vCJD presents with a progressive course of cognitive decline with prominent neuropsychiatric features often accompanied by sensory symptoms and leads to death after an average of 14 months. Transmission to humans occurs through ingestion of infected bovine meat products. There is no person-to-person transmission, but it can occur during invasive medical interventions. One of the characteristic features of prions is their resistance to a number of usual decontaminating procedures. Private room and other measures are not required for infection control. But for surgical procedures on any person with confirmed or suspected prion diseases, every effort should be made to plan carefully not only the procedure but also the infection prevention practices surrounding the procedure, e.g., instrument handling, storage, cleaning and decontamination, or disposal. Written protocols are essential.

Pathogenic Fungi and Their Modes of Transmission

Candida is a yeast that causes candidiasis. There are over 20 species of *Candida* that can cause infection in humans, the most common of which is *Candida albicans*. *Candida* can present on the skin and mucous membranes of humans without causing infection and is considered normal flora. However, overgrowth of these organisms is seen as collateral damage to the normal flora by antibiotic use or compromise of the immunity due to hematological malignancies, steroid use, and HIV infection. Symptoms range from local mucous membrane infections to widespread dissemination with multisystem organ failure.

Aspergillus is a mold. It is ubiquitous in nature and can exist in indoor and outdoor environments. Most people breathe in *Aspergillus* spores every day without being affected. The spectrum of illness includes allergic reactions, lung infections, and extrapulmonary dissemination. People who are at risk are patients with severe and prolonged neutropenia, receipt of high doses of glucocorticoids and other drugs, or conditions that lead to chronically impaired cellular immune responses.

Cryptococcus is yeast that can be found in soil throughout the world. People can inhale the yeast with no symptoms or mild pneumonia in immunocompetent patients. It is a common cause of meningoencephalitis in patients with HIV. Despite the finding of this fungus in pigeon guano, direct transmission from pigeons to humans has not been reported, neither has person-to-person transmission. Soil is the documented source of infection.

Endemic mycoses: Each of the four endemic mycoses, blastomycosis, histoplasmosis, coccidioidomycosis, and paracoccidioidomycosis, is geographically restricted to a specific area of the world. The fungi that cause coccidioidomycosis and histoplasmosis exist in the soil, while the fungi that cause blastomycosis and paracoccidioidomycosis are presumed to reside in nature, but their habitat has not been clearly identified. Each of these mycoses is caused by a thermally dimorphic fungus, and most infections are initiated in the lungs following inhalation of the conidia. Only few infections lead to disease which can be acute or chronic pneumonia or extra pulmonary. These mycoses are not transmissible among humans or other animals.

Tinea versicolor is a common superficial fungal infection caused by Malassezia which is a dimorphic fungus. Patients with this disorder often present with hypopigmented, hyperpigmented, or erythematous macules on the trunk and proximal upper extremities. Malassezia is a component of normal skin flora; transformation of Malassezia from yeast cells to a pathogenic mycelial form is associated with the development of clinical disease. External factors suspected of contributing to this conversion include exposure to hot and humid weather, hyperhidrosis, and the use of topical skin oils. Tinea versicolor is not transmitted from person to person and is not related to poor hygiene.

Cutaneous mycoses (ringworm or tinea) are caused by fungi that infect only the superficial keratinized tissue of the skin, hair, and nail. Three types of dermatophytes account for the majority of infections: *Epidermophyton*, *Trichophyton*, and *Microsporum*. Dermatophytoses have varied presentations and are named by the location involved, tinea capitis, tinea pedis, tinea corporis, and tinea cruris. Dermatophytes are classified as geophilic, zoophilic, or anthropophilic depending on whether their usual habitant is soil, animals, or humans. Dermatophytes are acquired by contact with contaminated soil or with infected humans or animals.

Sporotrichosis is a subacute to chronic infection caused by the dimorphic fungus Sporothrix schenckii. Infection usually involves cutaneous and subcutaneous tissues but can occasionally occur in other sites like lungs, meninges, and other viscera especially in individuals with underlying illnesses including alcoholism, diabetes mellitus, and AIDS. Days to weeks after cutaneous inoculation of the fungus, a papule develops at the site of inoculation. This primary lesion usually ulcerates, then similar lesions occur along lymphatic channels proximal to the original lesion. S. schenckii exists in wood, hay, and soil. Inhalation of S. schenckii from soil is the presumed route of transmission for pulmonary sporotrichosis. Zoonotic transmission is uncommon but has been traced back to a variety of animals, cats being the most common.

Pathogenic Parasites and Their Modes of Transmission

Parasites of medical importance come under the kingdom called Protista and Animalia. Protista includes the microscopic single-celled eukaryotes known as protozoa. In contrast, helminths are macroscopic, multicellular worms possessing well-differentiated tissues and complex organs and belong to the kingdom Animalia. Parasites are transmitted to humans through arthropod vector like plasmodia, babesia, *Trypanosoma,* and *Leishmania,* through the gastrointestinal tract like Giardia, Entamoeba histolytica, Isospora, Cyclospora, Toxoplasma, Cryptosporidium, Microsporidia, and Balantidium which typically will affect the gastrointestinal tract but can affect other organs as well. Some parasites are sexually transmitted like Trichomonas.

Protozoa

Plasmodium There are four species that normally infect humans, namely, *Plasmodium falciparum, Plasmodium vivax, Plasmodium ovale,* and *Plasmodium malariae.* Malaria is the most important parasitic disease of humans, with transmission in over 100 countries affecting close to three billion people and causing one to two million deaths each year [36]. The initial

symptoms and signs are nonspecific and may include tachycardia, tachypnea, chills, malaise, fatigue, diaphoresis, headache, cough, anorexia, nausea, vomiting, and diarrhea. Then periodic attacks of fever occur 48–72. Complications are due to severe anemia and capillary plugging from an adhesion of infected red blood cells with each other and endothelial lining of capillaries resulting in hypoxic injury to the brain and kidney. This occurs especially in *P. falciparum* infection where the parasitemia is more severe compared to the other species. Malaria is transmitted via the bite of a female Anopheles mosquito, which occurs mainly between dusk and dawn. Other comparatively rare mechanisms for transmission include congenitally acquired disease, blood transfusion, sharing of contaminated needles, and organ transplantation. In areas where malaria is endemic, the groups at high risk for severe malaria and its consequences include young children (6–36 months) and pregnant women. Older children and adults develop partial immunity after repeated infections and are at relatively low risk for severe disease. As disease incidence wanes, older age groups will become more susceptible due to decreasing immunity. Travelers to areas where malaria is endemic generally have no previous exposure to malaria parasites and are at very high risk for severe disease if infected. Modes of preventions include chemoprophylaxis and protection from mosquito bite by netting, protective clothing, and insect repellents which are also effective. Prompt diagnosis and treatment including "self-treatment" prevents complications.

Giardia lamblia has a worldwide distribution, particularly common in the tropics and subtropics. It can be asymptomatic but symptomatic giardiasis ranges from mild diarrhea to severe malabsorption syndrome. Usually, the onset of the disease is sudden and consists of foul smelling, watery diarrhea, abdominal cramps, flatulence, and steatorrhea. The life cycle consists of two stages, the trophozoite and the cyst. Transmission occurs by ingestion of the infective cyst. It is acquired through the consumption of inadequately treated contaminated water, ingestion of contaminated uncooked vegetables or fruits, and person-to-person spread by the fecal-oral route. The cyst stage is resistant to chlorine in concentrations used in most water treatment facilities. For prevention of transmission, asymptomatic reservoirs of infection should be identified and treated, contaminated food and water should be avoided, and drinking water from wells, lakes, and streams should be boiled, filtered, or iodine treated.

Entamoeba histolytica has a worldwide distribution. Although it is found in cold areas, the incidence is highest in tropical and subtropical regions that have poor sanitation and contaminated water. About 90 % of infections are asymptomatic, and the remaining produce a spectrum of clinical syndrome. Intestinal form causes diarrhea, flatulence, and cramping. In extraintestinal amebiasis, amebic abscesses are formed and the most common site is the liver. The main source of infection is water and food contamination. Symptomatic amebiasis is usually sporadic. The epidemic form is a result of direct person-to-person fecal-oral spread under conditions of poor personal hygiene. The essential measures for prevention are introduction of adequate sanitation measures, education about the routes of transmission, and avoidance in eating raw vegetables grown by sewage irrigation.

Other Protozoa

Protozoa/disease	Epidemiology and modes of transmission	Clinical manifestations	Prevention
Leishmania donovani/ Visceral leishmaniasis or kala-azar	Kala-azar occurs in three distinct epidemiologic patterns: 1. In the Mediterranean basin and parts of China and Russia, the reservoir hosts are primarily dogs and foxes. 2. In sub-Saharan Africa, rats and small carnivores are believed to be the main reservoirs. 3. In India and the neighboring countries (and Kenya), it is an anthroponosis (there is no other mammalian reservoir host other than human)	Symptoms begin with intermittent fever, weakness, diarrhea, and chills and sweating that may resemble malaria symptoms early in the infection. The organisms proliferate and invade cells of the liver, spleen, and bone marrow causing hepatosplenomegaly, weight loss, and anemia	Prompt treatment of human infections and control of reservoir hosts
			Protection from sand flies by screening and insect repellents
	The vector is the sand fly		
*L. tropica complex, L. aethiopica/*old world cutaneous leishmaniasis	*L. tropica* complex is present in many parts of Asia, Africa, and Europe	The first sign, a red papule, appears at the site of the fly's bite. This lesion becomes irritated with intense itching then enlarges and ulcerates	Prompt treatment and eradication of ulcers
	The urban form is thought to be an anthroponosis, while the rural form is zoonosis with human infections occurring only sporadically. The reservoir hosts are rodents	Gradually the ulcer becomes hard and crusted and exudes a thin, serous material	Control of sand flies and reservoir hosts
	L. aethiopica is endemic in Ethiopia and Kenya. The disease is a zoonosis with hyraxes serving as reservoir hosts		
	The vector is the sand fly		

(continued)

(continued)

Protozoa/disease	Epidemiology and modes of transmission	Clinical manifestations	Prevention
L. Mexican, L. braziliensis/New World cutaneous and mucocutaneous leishmaniasis	Occurs in South and Central America, especially in the Amazon basin	The types of lesions range from oriental sore to disseminated cutaneous leishmaniasis	Avoiding endemic areas
	Rodents, monkeys, raccoons, and domesticated dogs serve as reservoirs		Prompt treatment of infected individuals
	The vector is the sand fly		Control of sand flies and reservoir hosts
Trypanosoma brucei complex/African trypanosomiasis (sleeping sickness)	*T. brucei gambiense* is limited to tropical west and Central Africa	Sleeping sickness starts with an ulcer at the site of the fly bite. The disease progresses causing lethargy, tremors, and mental retardation. In the final stage the patient develop convulsions, and hemiplegia prior to death	Control of breeding sites of tsetse flies and use of insecticides
	An animal reservoir has not been proven for this infection		Treatment of human cases
	T. brucei rhodesiense is found primarily in East Africa, especially the cattle-raising countries		Avoiding insect bite by wearing protective clothing and using insect repellants
	Domestic animal hosts (cattle and sheep) and wild animals act as reservoir hosts		
	The vector is the tsetse fly		
Trypanosoma cruzi/American trypanosomiasis (Chagas' disease)	Found in South and Central America, wild animals are the reservoir hosts	May be asymptomatic. One of the earliest signs is development of erythematous and indurated area at the site of the insect bite	Insect control, eradication of nests
	The vector is the blood-sucking triatomine insects or kissing bugs	Accompanied with fever, myalgia, and fatigue	Treating infected person and exclusion of donors by screening blood
		The chronic disease is characterized by hepatosplenomegaly, myocarditis, and achalasia	
Balantidium coli/balantidiasis	*B. coli* is distributed worldwide	Mostly asymptomatic	Following good hygiene practices including washing all fruits and vegetables with clean water when preparing or eating them
	Swine and monkeys are the most important reservoirs	Symptomatic disease is characterized by abdominal pain, tenesmus, nausea, anorexia, and watery stools with blood and pus	
	Infections are transmitted by the fecal-oral route; outbreaks are associated with contamination of water supplies with pig feces	Extraintestinal invasion of organs is extremely rare in balantidiasis	
	Person-to-person spread has been implicated		

(continued)

(continued)

Protozoa/disease	Epidemiology and modes of transmission	Clinical manifestations	Prevention
Toxoplasma gondii/ toxoplasmosis	The definitive host is the domestic cat and other felines. Humans and other mammals are intermediate hosts. *T. gondii* is usually acquired by ingestion. Transplacental transmission from an infected mother to the fetus can occur. Human-to-human transmission, other than transplacental transmission, does not occur	After infecting the intestinal epithelium, the organisms spread to other organs especially the brain, lungs, liver, and eyes

Most primary infections in immunocompetent adults are asymptomatic. Encephalitis is the most common presentation of toxoplasmosis among AIDS patients. Congenital infection can result in abortion, stillbirth, or neonatal disease with encephalitis, chorioretinitis, and hepatosplenomegaly | Cooking food to safe temperature and avoiding drinking untreated water. Pregnant or immunocompromised. Avoid changing cat litter or wear disposable gloves and wash hands afterwards |
| *Cyclospora cayetanensis/* cyclosporiasis | Infection occurs worldwide

It is acquired by fecal-oral transmission, especially via contaminated water supplies. There is no evidence for an animal reservoir | An intestinal protozoan that causes watery diarrhea in both immunocompetent and immunocompromised individuals. The diarrhea can be prolonged and relapsing in immunocompromised patients | Avoiding food or water that may have been contaminated with feces

Chlorine or iodine is unlikely to kill *Cyclospora* oocysts |
| *Isospora belli/*isosporiasis | The organism is acquired by fecal-oral transmission of oocysts from either human or animal sources | An intestinal protozoan that causes diarrhea, especially in AIDS patients | Avoiding food or water that may have been contaminated with feces

Chlorine or iodine is unlikely to kill *Cyclospora* oocysts |
| *Cryptosporidium parvum/* cryptosporidiosis | The organism is acquired by fecal-oral transmission of oocysts from either human or animal sources

Water (drinking water and recreational water) is the most common method of transmission | The main symptom is diarrhea. It is most severe in AIDS patients | Practicing good hygiene

Avoid swimming if you are experiencing diarrhea and If infected, do not swim for at least 2 weeks after diarrhea stops |
| Microsporidia/ microsporidiosis | The organisms are transmitted by fecal-oral route. It is uncertain whether an animal reservoir exists | Causes severe, persistent, watery diarrhea in AIDS patients | Practicing good hygiene |
| *Trichomonas vaginalis/* trichomoniasis | This parasite has worldwide distribution, and sexual intercourse is the primary mode of transmission. Occasionally, infections can be transmitted by fomites (toilet articles and clothing)

Rarely infants may be infected by passage through the mother's infected birth canal | In women it can cause vaginitis with vaginal discharge and dysuria

In men it is mostly asymptomatic and very rarely may cause urethritis | Both male and female sex partners must be treated to avoid reinfection

Good personal hygiene, avoidance of shared toilet articles and clothing

Safe sexual practice |

Helminths

Helminths are multicellular organisms that cause morbidity and mortality worldwide. They cause different diseases in humans, but few helminthic infections cause life-threatening diseases. They enter the body through different routes including the mouth, skin, and the respiratory tract.

The helminths are classified into three major groups. These are as follows:
1. Trematodes (flukes)
2. Nematodes (round worms)
3. Cestodes (tapeworms)

Medically Important Trematodes (Flukes)

They are found in a wide range of habitats. The great majority inhabit the alimentary canal, liver, bile duct, ureter, and bladder of vertebrate animals.

Helminth/disease	Location in host	Epidemiology	Mode of transmission
Schistosoma haematobium/ schistosomiasis	The veins of the bladder of humans	Africa and the Middle East	Larva penetrates skin from snail-infected water
Schistosoma mansoni/ schistosomiasis	The veins of the intestine	Africa, South America, and the Middle East	Larva penetrates skin from snail-infected water
Fasciola hepatica/fascioliasis	Liver and bile duct	Worldwide	Aquatic vegetation
Paragonimus westermani/paragonimiasis	Lungs, brain, and other sites	Asia (China, India, Indonesia, Malaya, etc.) and some African countries	Raw crabs and other freshwater crustaceans

Medically Important Nematodes (Round Worms)

These helminths have a tough protective covering or cuticle. They have a complete digestive tract with both oral and anal openings. They are free-living (majority) or parasites of humans, plants, or animals. Their life cycle includes egg, larvae, and adult.

Helminth/disease	Location in host	Epidemiology	Mode of transmission
Ascaris lumbricoides/ ascariasis	Small intestine, larvae through lungs	Infecting more than 700 million people worldwide	Contaminated food and water
Ancylostoma duodenale/ hookworm infection	Small intestine, larvae through lungs	Temperate zones	From infected soils through skin
Necator americanus/ hookworm infection	Small intestine, larvae through lungs	Worldwide tropics and North America	From infected soils through skin
Ancylostoma braziliense/cutaneous larva migrans	Subcutaneous migratory larvae	Worldwide	Contact with soils contaminated by dog or cat feces
Toxocara canis and *Toxocara cati*/visceral larva migrans	Cerebral, myocardial, and pulmonary migratory larva	Worldwide	Ingesting soil contaminated by dog or cat feces
Strongyloides stercoralis/ strongyloidiasis	Duodenum, jejunum, and larva through skin and lungs	Worldwide	From infected soil through skin
Enterobius vermicularis (*pin worm*)/enterobiasis	Cecum, colon	Worldwide	Direct infection from a patient (fecal-oral route), self contamination

(continued)

(continued)

Helminth/disease	Location in host	Epidemiology	Mode of transmission
Trichuris trichiura (*whipworm*)/trichuriasis	Cecum, colon	Worldwide	Ingesting contaminated soils
Wuchereria bancrofti/ filariasis	Lymph nodes and the lymphatic vessels, microfilariae through the bloodstream	Infecting over 100 million people worldwide	Mosquito is the vector
Onchocerca volvulus/onchocerciasis	Skin, lymphatic vessels, and cornea; microfilariae through the subcutaneous tissue fluids	Africa and South America	Black fly is the vector
Loa loa/loiasis	Conjunctiva, microfilariae through the bloodstream	Western and Central Africa	Mango fly and deerfly are the vectors
Dracunculus medinensis/ dracunculiasis	Subcutaneous, usually leg and foot	India, Nile Valley, and Central, western, and equatorial Africa	Drinking contaminated water with
Trichinella spiralis/trichinellosis	Larvae in striated muscle	Worldwide, more than 100 different animal species can be infected	Consumption of undercooked pork
		But the main reservoir host for humans is swine	

Medically Important Cestodes (Tapeworms)

They require an intermediate host. Adult tapeworms inhabit the small intestine, where they live attached to the mucosa. Tapeworms do not have a digestive system. Their food is absorbed from the host's intestine.

Helminth	Location in host	Epidemiology	Mode of transmission
Hymenolepis nana (dwarf tapeworm)/hymenolepiasis	Small intestine	Worldwide	Consumption of contaminated raw vegetables, direct infection from a patient (fecal-oral route), and self contamination
Hymenolepis diminuta (rat tapeworm)/hymenolepiasis	Small intestine	Worldwide, humans and rats are the reservoir	Ingestion of food contaminated by rat flea
Echinococcus granulosus (dog tapeworm)/ echinococcosis (hydatidosis)	Larvae in the liver, lung, brain, peritoneum, long bone, and kidney	Worldwide, definitive hosts are dogs where worms live in small intestine. Humans are intermediate host carrying the hydatid cyst (larva)	Ingestion of food contaminated by feces of dogs, handling or caressing infected dogs
Taenia saginata (beef tapeworm)/taeniasis	Small intestine	Worldwide	Undercooked beef
Taenia solium (pork tapeworm)/taeniasis	Small intestine	Worldwide	Undercooked pork
Diphyllobothrium latum (broad or fish tapeworm)/ diphyllobothriasis	Small intestine	Worldwide	Undercooked freshwater fish

References

1. Kluytmans J, van Belkum A, Verbrugh H. Nasal carriage of *Staphylococcus aureus*: epidemiology, underlying mechanisms, and associated risks. Clin Microbiol Rev. 1997;10(3):505–20.
2. Chu VH, Woods CW, Miro JM, Hoen B, Cabell CH, Pappas PA, Federspiel J, Athan E, Stryjewski ME, Nacinovich F, Marco F, Levine DP, Elliott TS, Fortes CQ, Tornos P, Gordon DL, Utili R, Delahaye F, Corey GR, Fowler Jr VG, International Collaboration on Endocarditis-Prospective Cohort Study Group. Emergence of coagulase-negative staphylococci as a cause of native valve endocarditis. Clin Infect Dis. 2008;46(2):232–42.
3. Pfaller MA, Herwaldt LA. Laboratory, clinical, and epidemiological aspects of coagulase-negative staphylococci. Clin Microbiol Rev. 1988;1(3):281–99.
4. Schrag SJ, Zywicki S, Farley MM, Reingold AL, Harrison LH, Lefkowitz LB, Hadler JL, Danila R, Cieslak PR, Schuchat A. Group B streptococcal disease in the era of intrapartum antibiotic prophylaxis. N Engl J Med. 2000;342(1):15–20.
5. Hidron AI, Edwards JR, Patel J, Horan TC, Sievert DM, Pollock DA, Fridkin SK, National Healthcare Safety Network Team; Participating National Healthcare Safety Network Facilities. NHSN annual update: antimicrobial-resistant pathogens associated with healthcare-associated infections: annual summary of data reported to the National Healthcare Safety Network at the Centers for Disease Control and Prevention, 2006–2007. Infect Control Hosp Epidemiol. 2008;29(11):996–1011.
6. Hopkins RS, Jajosky RA, Hall PA, Adams DA, Connor FJ, Sharp P, Anderson WJ, Fagan RF, Aponte JJ, Nitschke DA, Worsham CA, Adekoya N, Chang MH, Centers for Disease Control and Prevention (CDC). Summary of notifiable diseases–United States, 2003. MMWR Morb Mortal Wkly Rep. 2005;52(54):1–85.
7. Weber DJ, Saviteer SM, Rutala WA, Thomann CA. Clinical significance of *Bacillus* species isolated from blood cultures. South Med J. 1989;82(6):705–9.
8. Kalapothaki V, Sapounas T, Xirouchaki E, Papoutsakis G, Trichopoulos D. Prevalence of diphtheria carriers in a population with disappearing clinical diphtheria. Infection. 1984;12(6):387–9.
9. Scallan E, Hoekstra RM, Angulo FJ, Tauxe RV, Widdowson MA, Roy SL, Jones JL, Griffin PM. Foodborne illness acquired in the United States–major pathogens. Emerg Infect Dis. 2011;17(1):7–15.
10. Lerner PI. The lumpy jaw. Cervicofacial actinomycosis. Infect Dis Clin North Am. 1988;2(1):203–20.
11. Kwartler JA, Limaye A. Pathologic quiz case 1. Cervicofacial actinomycosis. Arch Otolaryngol Head Neck Surg. 1989;115(4):524–7.
12. Vaneechoutte M, Verschraegen G, Claeys G, Weise B, Van den Abeele AM. Respiratory tract carrier rates of *Moraxella* (Branhamella) catarrhalis in adults

and children and interpretation of the isolation of *M. catarrhalis* from sputum. J Clin Microbiol. 1990;28(12):2674–80.
13. Bennish ML, et al. Potentially lethal complications of shigellosis. Rev Infect Dis. 1991;13 Suppl 4:S319–24.
14. Keusch GT, Formal SB, Bennish ML. Shigellosis. In: Warren KS, Mahmoud AAF, editors. Tropical and geographical medicine. New York: McGraw-Hill; 1990. p. 763.
15. Hohmann EL. Nontyphoidal salmonellosis. Clin Infect Dis. 2001;32(2):263–9.
16. Warburton DW, Bowen B, Konkle A. The survival and recovery of *Pseudomonas aeruginosa* and its effect upon salmonellae in water: methodology to test bottled water in Canada. Can J Microbiol. 1994;40(12):987–92.
17. Silverman AR, Nieland ML. Hot tub dermatitis: a familial outbreak of *Pseudomonas folliculitis*. J Am Acad Dermatol. 1983;8(2):153–6.
18. Goel N, Wattal C, Oberoi JK, Raveendran R, Datta S, Prasad KJ. Trend analysis of antimicrobial consumption and development of resistance in non-fermenters in a tertiary care hospital in Delhi, India. J Antimicrob Chemother. 2011;66:1625–30.
19. Bosilkovski M, Dimzova M, Grozdanovski K. Natural history of brucellosis in an endemic region in different time periods. Acta Clin Croat. 2009;48(1):41–6.
20. Güriş D, Strebel PM, Bardenheier B, Brennan M, Tachdjian R, Finch E, Wharton M, Livengood JR. Changing epidemiology of pertussis in the United States: increasing reported incidence among adolescents and adults, 1990–1996. Clin Infect Dis. 1999;28(6):1230–7.
21. Pertussis—United States, 1997–2000. Centers for disease control and prevention (CDC). MMWR Morb Mortal Wkly Rep. 2002;51(4):73–6.
22. Ward JI, Cherry JD, Chang SJ, Partridge S, Lee H, Treanor J, Greenberg DP, Keitel W, Barenkamp S, Bernstein DI, Edelman R, Edwards K, APERT Study Group. Efficacy of an acellular pertussis vaccine among adolescents and adults. N Engl J Med. 2005;353(15):1555–63.
23. Luby JP. Pneumonia caused by *Mycoplasma pneumoniae* infection. Clin Chest Med. 1991;12(2):237–44.
24. Mahajan SK, Rolain JM, Sankhyan N, Kaushal RK, Raoult D. Pediatric scrub typhus in Indian Himalayas. Indian J Pediatr. 2008;75(9):947–9.
25. Vivekanandan M, Mani A, Priya YS, Singh AP, Jayakumar S, Purty S. Outbreak of scrub typhus in Pondicherry. J Assoc Phys India. 2010;58:24–8.
26. Narvencar KP, Rodrigues S, Nevrekar RP, Dias L, Dias A, Vaz M, Gomes E. Scrub typhus in patients reporting with acute febrile illness at a tertiary health care institution in Goa. Indian J Med Res. 2012;136(6):1020–4.
27. Gurung S, Pradhan J, Bhutia PY. Outbreak of scrub typhus in the North East Himalayan region-Sikkim: an emerging threat. Indian J Med Microbiol. 2013;31(1):72–4.

28. Sepkowitz KA. How contagious is tuberculosis? Clin Infect Dis. 1996;23(5):954–62.

29. Truman RW, Singh P, Sharma R, Busso P, Rougemont J, Paniz-Mondolfi A, Kapopoulou A, Brisse S, Scollard DM, Gillis TP, Cole ST. Probable zoonotic leprosy in the southern United States. N Engl J Med. 2011; 364(17):1626–33.

30. Karonga Prevention Trial Group. Randomised controlled trial of single BCG, repeated BCG, or combined BCG and killed *Mycobacterium leprae* vaccine for prevention of leprosy and tuberculosis in Malawi. Lancet. 1996;348(9019):17–24.

31. Robertson SE, Featherstone DA, Gacic-Dobo M, Hersh BS. Rubella and congenital rubella syndrome: global update. Rev Panam Salud Publica. 2003;14(5):306–15.

32. Gupta RK, Best J, MacMahon E. Mumps and the UK epidemic 2005. BMJ. 2005;330(7500):1132–5.

33. Jernigan JA, Lowry BS, Hayden FG, Kyger SA, Conway BP, Gröschel DH, Farr BM. Adenovirus type 8 epidemic keratoconjunctivitis in an eye clinic: risk factors and control. J Infect Dis. 1993;167(6):1307–13.

34. Lyons A, Longfield J, Kuschner R, Straight T, Binn L, Seriwatana J, Reitstetter R, Froh IB, Craft D, McNabb K, Russell K, Metzgar D, Liss A, Sun X, Towle A, Sun W. A double-blind, placebo-controlled study of the safety and immunogenicity of live, oral type 4 and type 7 adenovirus vaccines in adults. Vaccine. 2008;26(23):2890–8.

35. Liaw YF, Tsai SL, Sheen IS, Chao M, Yeh CT, Hsieh SY, Chu CM. Clinical and virological course of chronic hepatitis B virus infection with hepatitis C and D virus markers. Am J Gastroenterol. 1998;93(3):354–9.

36. Filler S, Causer LM, Newman RD, et al. Malaria surveillance–United States, 2001. MMWR Surveill Summ. 2003;52:1–14.

Part II

Vaccinations and Infection Prevention

Vaccinations and Infection Prevention

Vivek Kak

The hospital environment is a unique example of an enclosed environment where two distinct groups of individuals interact. The close interactions between health-care workers and the patients' that they take care for act as a two-way street where pathogens can transfer rarely from the patient to the health-care workers (HCW) and more commonly from the health-care workers to the patient. The aim of infection prevention in this setting is to minimize and attempt to eliminate this two-way traffic and thus keep the health-care worker safe and healthy from patient-acquired infections and as importantly prevent transfer of pathogenic organism and infections from the health-care worker to the patient.

The risk of acquisition of an infection by the HCW during their work can be minimized by the strict adherence to basic principles of infection prevention including (1) strict hand hygiene while taking care of patients, (2) rapid institution of appropriate isolation precautions for patients with suspected infections, and (3) the use of vaccinations appropriately among health-care worker [1]. This chapter discusses the role of vaccinations among health-care workers both to prevent the occupational acquisition of vaccine-preventable diseases by HCW and prevent the HCW acting as vector for dissemination of disease within the hospital setting.

The use of vaccination as modality for infection prevention was probably the most important public health achievement of the twentieth century. The appropriate use of vaccines has led to the elimination of infections such as smallpox as well as the decrease and virtual elimination of infections such as poliomyelitis. It is important to ensure that HCW are immune to vaccine-preventable diseases at the time of hire. The use of appropriate vaccines among HCW can lead to prevention of transmission of these infections and also lead to decreased absenteeism among the personnel. This "ounce" of prevention is much more cost-effective than managing outbreaks of vaccine-preventable diseases if they occur among health-care workers.

General Guidelines

The Center for Diseases Control (CDC), USA, and Advisory Committee on Immunization Practices (ACIP) have published general guidelines about the use of vaccines among health-care workers [2].

The general principles for these should focus on:

- Appropriate screening of new hires for immunity to vaccine-preventable diseases prior to them reporting for work and reviewing immunity status on a regular basis.
- Vaccinations needed by HCW should be provided free of charge by the institution.
- Mandatory vaccination programs should be considered as they increase vaccination rates

V. Kak, M.D. (✉)
Allegiance Health, 1100East Michigan Avenue, #305, Jackson, MI 49201, USA
e-mail: vkak@yahoo.com

among HCW to much greater extent than voluntary programs.

- Immunocompromised and pregnant employees require special consideration in the provision of vaccinations.
- The screening and immunization records of the HCW should be maintained in the HCW medical record in the occupational health department.

The vaccination of HCW can be divided into vaccinations based on the job classification of the HCW [1–3]. All health-care workers should be immune to varicella, measles, mumps, and rubella. The HCW who have the potential for exposure to blood or other body fluids should be immunized against hepatitis B. Recent guidelines in the USA and mandates from licensing organisms have suggested that HCW with direct patient contact should be immunized against influenza and pertussis [2, 4]. Laboratory personnel as well as select health-care workers in special circumstances should also be offered vaccinations against meningococcal diseases, poliomyelitis, as well as *Salmonella typhi*. In areas of endemic diseases or in special conditions, HCW may benefit from hepatitis A and rabies vaccination. All HCW should also be recommended vaccinations based on age and other comorbid conditions such as the pneumococcal and tetanus-diphtheria vaccination [2].

HCW who are immunocompromised need special attention, as they should not be vaccinated with live vaccinations such as the measles-mumps-rubella vaccine and the varicella vaccine [5]. Based on the nature of their immunosuppression, they may require vaccination such as the pneumococcal, Haemophilus influenza type b, and meningococcal vaccines. Pregnant HCW also require special consideration since generally live attenuated vaccines are contraindicated in pregnancy. It is thus of utmost importance the female HCW of childbearing age be screened prior to pregnancy for certain vaccine-preventable diseases especially rubella and varicella. If the female HCW have no clinical or serological evidence of these diseases, they should be offered immunization against these diseases especially based on the severe consequences of developing either rubella or chickenpox during pregnancy [1, 2, 5, 6].

If vaccines are offered to the HCW, a detailed evaluation of the HCW should be done to ensure that there is no contraindication for any vaccine. In the presence of absolute contraindications, the vaccine should not be offered, but a detailed discussion with the HCW should be done discussing risk of the disease and also whether reassignment of job duties may be an option. It should be noted the most common contraindication tends to be the presence of an anaphylactic reaction to a previous dose of the vaccine or a vaccine component. The development of low-grade fevers, mild local tenderness, a history of allergies, or family histories of allergies or seizures are not contraindications for vaccination [5, 6].

Tables 2.1 and 2.2 list the vaccines recommended for health-care workers.

Individual Vaccines

Strongly Recommended Vaccines

Hepatitis B Vaccine

Infections due to blood-borne pathogens such as hepatitis B virus (HBV), hepatitis C virus, and HIV are a major occupational hazard for HCW. The risk of acquisition of these diseases can be decreased by institution of universal precautions, use of preventive measures such as using needleless devices and, in the case of hepatitis B, universal use of the hepatitis B vaccine and postexposure prophylaxis using HBIG (hepatitis B immunoglobulin) if indicated. The use of the above multimodal approach has led to a decrease in HBV in the USA among HCW from 17,000 cases in 1983 to 400 in 1995 [7].

The risk of acquiring HBV among HCW is related to occupational exposure of HCW percutaneous or mucosal surfaces to blood or body fluids containing HBV especially fluids that also contain HBeAntigen (HBeAg) which is a marker for active viral replication and a higher viral load [8]. The risk of disease transmission of HBV during percutaneous exposure is thought to be between 6 % and 30 % and is much higher in this setting compared to mucosal exposure to the virus [8]. The transmission of HBV has also been

Table 2.1 Vaccines recommended strongly for health-care workers

Vaccine	Indication	Schedule and booster in nonimmune individuals	Precautions/contraindications
Hepatitis B	All health-care workers	Series of 3 IM injections given at 0, 1, and 6 months, repeat series if nonresponder: no booster	Avoid if anaphylaxis to baker's yeast
Varicella	All health-care workers	A series of 2 injections given 4 weeks apart	Pregnancy/immunocompromised state/anaphylaxis to neomycin or gelatin/avoid aspirin for 6 weeks after vaccination/recent use of immunoglobulin
Influenza	All health-care workers	Yearly injections	Anaphylaxis to eggs/avoid live vaccine if working with patients who have received stem cell transplants
Measles	All health-care workers	Series of 2 injections given 4 weeks apart	Pregnancy/immunocompromised state/anaphylaxis to neomycin or gelatin/recent use of immunoglobulin
Mumps	All health-care workers	Series of 2 injections given 4 weeks apart	Pregnancy/immunocompromised state/anaphylaxis to neomycin or gelatin/recent use of immunoglobulin
Rubella	All health-care workers	Single injection with no booster	Pregnancy/immunocompromised state/anaphylaxis to neomycin or gelatin/recent use of immunoglobulin
Pertussis	All health-care workers	Since injection with the acellular vaccine (Tdap)	History of encephalopathy, Guillain-Barre syndrome <6 weeks after a dose of tetanus toxoid vaccine or a progressive neurological disease. Age is not a contraindication among HCW

Source: Adapted from Ref. [1]

associated with contaminated medical instruments and is a particular problem among hemodialysis centers. The CDC has published guidelines for prevention of HBV in the dialysis setting, stressing monthly testing of HBsAg among susceptible patients, immunization of all susceptible hemodialysis patients with the HBV vaccine, isolating patients with chronic hepatitis B, and not sharing any equipments and supplies among patients [9]. The HBV vaccine however has a diminished response among hemodialysis patients, and thus a higher dose and booster doses may be indicated among hemodialysis patients [10].

Preexposure Prophylaxis

The HBV vaccine in generally administered in a three dose vaccine series at 0-, 1- and 6-month schedules. The efficacy of the vaccine is >90 % after the third dose in terms of formation of a protective antibody titer. The vaccine should be given in the deltoid area since gluteal injection leads to poor immunogenicity. All HCW should have an anti-HBs antibody titer checked around

2 months after the third dose of the vaccine; if they do not have a protective titer of ≥ 10 mIU, they should get revaccinated with a repeat series of the vaccine. Around 50 % of individuals who did not respond to the first series of the HBV vaccine respond to the second series of the vaccine. If the HCW does not respond to the second series, they should be labeled as a nonresponder. It is also important to test these individuals for HBsAntigen (HBsAg) in case they are not already infected with hepatitis B [2].

There are currently two single antigen hepatitis B vaccine, Recombivax HB (Merck) and Engerix-B (GSK), and a combined hepatitis A and hepatitis B vaccine, Twinrix (GSK). The single antigen HBV vaccines are interchangeable and either can be used to finish the series; however, the vaccination series does not need to be restarted if the second or third dose is delayed. The major contraindication for immunization with HBV is a history of hypersensitivity to yeast or any other vaccine component. The presence of autoimmune disease, pregnancy, and history of

Table 2.2 Vaccines recommended in special circumstances

Vaccine	Indication	Schedule and booster	Precaution/contraindication
Hepatitis A	Travel to area with disease or work in hospitals with high rates of exposure	Two doses of the vaccine given at least 6 months apart	History of anaphylaxis to first dose/use in pregnancy only if high risk of disease
Typhoid	Travel to area with disease or work in hospitals with high rates of exposure: laboratory workers who frequently work with *Salmonella typhi*	Single dose of the injectable vaccine with boosters every 2 years or four doses of the oral Ty21a vaccine given on alternate days with a booster series every 5 years	Avoid oral vaccine in pregnancy and in immunocompromised HCW; avoid oral vaccine in HCW involved in direct patient care
Meningococcal	Travel to area with disease or work in hospitals with high rates of exposure: laboratory workers who frequently work with *Neisseria meningitidis*	Single dose with boosters every 5 years	Use polysaccharide vaccine if HCW >55 years
Polio	Travel to area with disease or work in hospitals with high rates of exposure: laboratory workers who frequently work with specimens that may contain polioviruses	Single dose of the injectable polio vaccine (IPV) if previously immunized; if unimmunized that three doses with the second 4–8 weeks after the first and the last 6–12 months after the second	Avoid in pregnancy unless high risk and if anaphylaxis to streptomycin or neomycin
Pneumococcal	HCW with chronic medical problems	Use the Prevnar 13 conjugate vaccine in immunocompromised HCW followed by the pneumococcal polysaccharide vaccine 8 weeks later	Use single dose of polysaccharide vaccine if not immunocompromised
Rabies	HCW who take care of patients with rabies	Preexposure use on days 0,7, 21, or 28 (human diploid cell vaccine); postexposure booster may be required despite previous vaccination	Postexposure prophylaxis should follow guidelines including use of rabies immunoglobulin

Source: Adapted from Ref. [1]

Guillain-Barre syndrome are not contraindications to the receipt of the vaccine.

Postexposure Prophylaxis

If the unimmunized or a nonresponder HCW sustains a needle-stick injury from a patient with evidence of chronic HBV as evidenced by presence of HBsAntigen, they should be given HBIG (hepatitis B hyperimmune globulin) within 7 days and preferably within 24 h and should simultaneously reinitiate the three-dose hepatitis B vaccination, if the HCW did not previously finish the second hepatitis B series [2, 11]. If the HCW has had two series of the HBV vaccine and was still a nonresponder, they should receive a second dose of HBIG, 1 month after the first dose [2].

Table 2.3 lists the postexposure prophylaxis for HCW exposed to hepatitis B.

Varicella Vaccine

Varicella-zoster virus (VZV) is seen in the hospital setting either as primary infection with chickenpox or more often in the adult setting as zoster, either dermatomal zoster or rarely disseminated zoster. The virus is highly contagious among susceptible hosts and can lead to high morbidity as well as mortality among immunocompromised individuals, pregnant women, and in neonates. Susceptible HCW are often exposed to VZV while taking care of patients with either dermatomal zoster, disseminated zoster, or chickenpox. They can also acquire the infection from visitors or other staff, and nosocomial transmission most

Table 2.3 Post exposure prophylaxis for hepatitis B

HCW vaccination/ serostatus	Source HBs-Antigen positive	Source HBs-Antigen negative	Source unknown
Unvaccinated	Hepatitis B immunoglobulin (HBIG) and initiate vaccination	Vaccination alone	Vaccination alone
Responder to vaccine	No treatment	No treatment	No treatment
Nonresponder after one series	HBIG and reinitiate vaccination	No treatment	If high-risk source: HBIG and revaccination
Nonresponder after two series	HBIG given twice with the doses separated by one month	No treatment	HBIG given twice with the doses separated by one month
Unknown response	Test for anti-HBs: If $\geq$10 Miu/mL: no treatment If <10 Miu/mL: HBIG and vaccination	No treatment	Test for anti-HBs: If $\geq$10 Miu/mL: no treatment If <10 Miu/mL: HBIG and vaccination

Source: Adapted from Ref. [2]

often occurs because of a lag in diagnosis and a delay in instituting proper infection control precautions [12, 13]. The CDC suggests that only patients with chickenpox or disseminated zoster be placed in airborne and contact precautions; however, VZV DNA can be found in the throat even in patients with dermatomal zoster, and there have been nosocomial outbreaks of VZV due to patients with dermatomal zoster who were in appropriate contact isolation [14]. Only HCW with evidence of immunity to varicella should take care of patients with suspected/confirmed varicella or dermatomal or disseminated zoster [1, 2, 15, 16].

Preexposure Prophylaxis

It is important to ensure that all HCW are immune to varicella. This can be documented by serological testing for VZV or with a history of typical varicella especially for individuals born before 1998. HCW who are not immune to varicella should get two dose of the varicella vaccine administered at least 4–8 weeks apart. The vaccine series does not need to be restarted if the second dose is >8 weeks after the first. The vaccine should not be use in pregnant HCW or HCW with HIV or severe immunosuppression. HCW generally do not require any work restriction after vaccination; however, if they develop a vaccine-related rash after vaccination, they should avoid contact with patients/individuals who are susceptible to varicella [16].

Postexposure Prophylaxis

All HCW potentially exposed to varicella should be identified as soon after exposure and evaluated to see if they are immune or susceptible to varicella. HCW who have serological evidence of immunity or those who have had two doses of the vaccine should be considered immune but told to monitor for any symptoms suggestive of varicella daily between days 8 and 21 after exposure. Exposed HCW who only received a single dose of the vaccine should get the second dose within 3–5 days after exposure and then monitored as above. If they did not receive the second dose or if it was delayed >5 days after exposure, they should be furloughed from duty from days 8 to 21 postexposure [2, 3].

Nonimmune HCW who are exposed to varicella need to be furlonged from work from days 8 to 21 after exposure as they are potentially infective during this period. They should also receive postexposure vaccination generally within 3–5 days after exposure as long as no contraindications exist to vaccination. If the HCW is at risk of severe disease due to varicella and vaccination is contraindicated (e.g., pregnancy or HIV), varicella-zoster immune globulin (VZIG) should be considered. It should be given within 72 h after exposure and is dosed at 12.5 U/kg intramuscularly with a maximum dose of 625 U. VZIG can prolong the incubation period for varicella, and therefore all HCW who get VZIG should be furlonged till day 28 after exposure [2].

Influenza Vaccine

Seasonal outbreaks of influenza are a major cause of hospitalizations among patients in the USA. In India, limited influenza activity occurs all year around with increased activity observed during rains [17]. HCW are exposed to influenza in the workplace and thus are at risk of acquiring influenza as well as transmitting influenza to patients and other HCW. The development of influenza or influenza-like illness by HCW leads to significant absenteeism among HCW. Influenza often causes nosocomial outbreaks of respiratory illness among hospitalized individuals and can lead to increased morbidity and mortality in patients. The use of annual influenza vaccination among HCW has been shown to lead to a decrease in absenteeism among HCW due to respiratory illnesses [18]. It also has been shown that high rates of influenza vaccination among HCW can lead to decreased morbidity and mortality due to all causes and deaths from pneumonia in patients [19, 20]. These data have led to proposals of mandatory annual vaccination of HCW against influenza [21]. The influenza vaccine efficacy varies on yearly basis based on the "match" between the vaccine strains and the circulating community strains of influenza. Annual influenza vaccination is recommended, as the postvaccination immunity wanes over time and circulating influenza strains often change season to season.

Preexposure Prophylaxis

The influenza vaccine is recommended in the USA for all persons over 6 months of age who have no medical contraindication. It has become mandatory in a growing number of health-care institutions in the USA. HCW should receive the vaccine as soon as the vaccine is available and prior to the start of the influenza season in their community. There are two types of influenza vaccine available, the trivalent inactivated vaccine (TIV) and the live attenuated intranasal vaccine (LAIV). The TIV can be administered to any individual >6 months of age intramuscularly, while the LAIV is only licensed for use in healthy nonpregnant individuals between 2 and 49 years of age. HCW should not receive LAIV if they have close contact with severely immunocompromised hospitalized patients such as those with stem cell transplants. The main contraindication to annual influenza vaccination is hypersensitivity to eggs or any component of the vaccine [2].

Postexposure Prophylaxis

HCW should be strongly encouraged to use influenza vaccinations if there is community or nosocomial outbreak of influenza. If an unimmunized HCW is exposed to a patient with influenza, they should be immunized with TIV and offered chemoprophylaxis with either oseltamivir or zanamivir used one dose daily for 10 days postexposure. It is also important to limit contact between patients being treated for influenza and other individuals to minimize the spread of drug-resistant virus from patients [2, 3, 5].

Measles, Mump, and Rubella (MMR) Vaccine

Measles, mumps, and rubella are all highly contagious viral illnesses whose incidence has decreased in developing countries due to the widespread use of the MMR vaccine. Though rare, these three diseases are an important risk for HCW as all three can be transmitted through the droplet route. They can and are often transmitted by individuals prior to developing symptoms [22]. With the decreased incidence of clinical disease by these three viruses, often health-care providers may not recognize the symptoms of these diseases, and this may lead to late institution of proper infection prevention precautions and thus exposure of HCW to these viruses [23, 24]. There have been health-care-associated cases of measles, as well as mumps and rubella. HCW are often at a greater risk of developing measles as infected persons often seek medical care because of the severity of disease [24]. The outbreak of these viruses in the hospital setting is multifactorial and often is due to (1) inadequate utilization of precautions for suspected patients which mainly consist of droplet precautions for mumps and rubella while in the case of measles include both droplet and airborne precautions, (2) lack of immunity to these viruses in a substantial minority of HCW who feel they are immune and thus fail to take appropriate precautions, and (3) lack of mandatory vaccinations or documentation of immunity leading to susceptible HCW who may propagate the disease. The development to disease due to these viruses is often traumatic to HCW as seen in cases of rubella among pregnant HCW which can lead to congenital abnormalities in up to 90 % of women who get infected in their first trimester [3].

Preexposure Prophylaxis

All HCW should demonstrate evidence of immunity to measles, mumps, and rubella prior to reporting for clinical duty. This can be either serologically, the laboratory confirmation of disease, birth before 1957 (except for rubella), or receipt of two doses of the MMR vaccine (only one required for rubella). In the absence of documentation of the above criteria, it is recommended that HCW get two doses of the MMR vaccine given 4 weeks apart for measles and mumps. In the case of lack of immunity to rubella, only one dose of the MMR vaccine is required. The MMR vaccine is a live virus vaccine and has been associated with rare side effects mainly in children. These rare side effects include anaphylaxis, acute arthritis (due to the rubella component), and thrombocytopenia. The vaccine should not be given to pregnant females and HCW with severe immunosuppression. Female HCW should also be counseled to avoid becoming pregnant for 4 weeks after getting the MMR vaccine. There is no need to restrict recently MMR-vaccinated HCW in terms of job duties [2, 5].

Postexposure Prophylaxis

The key to postexposure prophylaxis among HCW to these three viruses is to avoid exposure. Thus rapid institution of appropriate precautions is the key to avoid health-care acquisition of disease. HCW should follow appropriate respiratory precautions regardless of their immunity status. Nonimmune HCW who are exposed to measles should be offered the first dose of the MMR vaccine within the first 72 h after exposure and furlonged from work from day 5 to 21 after exposure. Those HCW who have had one but not two doses of vaccine can remain at work but should

get the second dose of the vaccine. Postexposure prophylaxis can also be provided to HCW by the use of intramuscular immune globulin at the dose of 0.25 ml/kg but must be given within 6 days of exposure. HCW who receive immune globulin should be furlonged from work from day 5 to 28 postexposure.

Pertussis Vaccine

Pertussis is a highly contagious bacterial illness whose incidence has been increasing in the recent years most likely due to the waning immunity following immunization with the diphtheria toxoid, tetanus toxoid, and acellular pertussis (DTaP) vaccine. Among adults the disease mainly presents as protracted cough; however, susceptible infants especially those too young to be vaccinated are at a high risk of severe disease especially hospitalization and death [25]. These susceptible infants are generally infected by adult or adolescents whose immunity from childhood vaccinations has waned. Health-care-associated outbreaks of pertussis have occurred from patients to HCW as well from HCW to patients mainly because of the presence of waned immunity among HCW as well as failure to recognize disease among HCW and patients and take appropriate isolation precautions or furlong symptomatic HCW and then provide prophylaxis (if needed) and treatment [26, 27].

Preexposure Prophylaxis

All HCW regardless of age should receive a single dose of tetanus toxoid, diphtheria toxoid, and acellular pertussis (Tdap) vaccine. The use of this vaccine among all HCW will protect them against pertussis and is also expected to lead to decreased transmission from the HCW to patients, family members, and the community. At the current time Tdap is only licensed for a single dose, and future vaccinations of HCW after 10 years should utilize the tetanus toxoid diphtheria toxoid vaccine (Td) [2].

Postexposure Prophylaxis

All HCW exposed to patients with pertussis should be offered chemoprophylaxis especially if they work with pregnant women or neonates [27].

The receipt of Tdap does not preclude using chemoprophylaxis among exposed HCW. If the HCW has not received Tdap, they should be immunized alongside being offered chemoprophylaxis. The drug of choice for prophylaxis is a 5-day once-daily course of azithromycin. In HCW who are allergic to macrolides, trimethoprim-sulphamethoxazole is the preferred alternative.

Vaccines Recommended in Special Circumstances

Hepatitis A Vaccine
In the USA, the incidence of hepatitis A virus (HAV) infection has diminished drastically with the introduction of the HAV vaccine. In the USA, HCW are not thought to be a higher risk for HAV diseases; however, nosocomial outbreaks of HAV have occurred especially when the source patient was not jaundiced or had diarrhea [28]. In areas of the world where HAV is more common, HCW may have a higher risk of acquisition of HAV compared to the USA. The HAV vaccine is generally given intramuscularly in two doses given at least 6 months apart.

Preexposure Prophylaxis
The current immunization schedule in the USA recommends the HAV vaccine for all children; however, the HAV vaccine is not recommended routinely for HCW. However, HCW in areas of high incidence of HAV or who travel to these areas should consider getting the HAV vaccine [2].

Postexposure Prophylaxis
HCW who are exposed to HAV can be offered postexposure prophylaxis using immunoglobulin (IG). When administered within 2 weeks of exposure to hepatitis A, IG is 85–90 % effective in preventing disease. This protection involves IG preventing early disease, while the subclinical viremia from the exposure providing long-lasting immunity. The dose of IG for postexposure prophylaxis is 0.02 mg/kg. Since 1995 postexposure prophylaxis can also be administered using the hepatitis A vaccine, and thus these days IG use for postexposure prophylaxis is generally recom-mended for those individuals who cannot be vaccinated because of age (less than 12 months), those with an allergy to the vaccine components, or those who refuse vaccination [29].

Typhoid Vaccine
The incidence of typhoid fever has declined in the USA, and majority of the cases generally occur in individuals who report foreign travel. However, laboratory-acquired typhoid fever has been reported in the USA among individuals working in the microbiology laboratory [30]. In areas of high incidence of typhoid fever, HCW may be at higher risk of acquiring this disease as it has been shown to transmit *Salmonella typhi* nosocomially via the hands of infected persons. It is recommended that microbiologist and those HCW who work frequently with *Salmonella typhi* should be vaccinated against the disease. There are currently two licensed typhoid vaccines: the oral live attenuated Ty21a vaccine and the intramuscular capsular polysaccharide vaccine. The protective efficacy of both these vaccines is around 50–80 %. The oral vaccine is given in a series of four capsules taken on alternative days and provides immunity for 5 years. The single intramuscular vaccine needs a booster every 2 years. The live oral vaccine should not be used in immunocompromised individuals.

Meningococcal Vaccine
Meningococcal disease is rare among HCW; however, nosocomial transmission of *Neisseria meningitidis* has occurred in HCW who work in the laboratory setting or who have had contact with the respiratory secretions of infected individuals [31]. The prophylactic use of the meningococcal vaccines is generally recommended for HCW who have repeated contact with isolates of *Neisseria meningitidis* especially those working in clinical laboratories where *Neisseria meningitidis* is frequently encountered or those HCW who have functional asplenia or with persistent complement component deficiencies or HIV [2, 5]. The conjugate meningococcal vaccine is generally recommended for HCW, and HCW should be immunized every 5 years if they remain in a high risk group or environment.

Postexposure Prophylaxis

Postexposure prophylaxis for HCW exposed to meningococcal disease is indicated if the HCW had intensive, unprotected contact with infected patients. This includes unprotected contact during mouth-to-mouth resuscitation, endotracheal intubation, or endotracheal tube management. HCW who have been vaccinated still need prophylaxis with antimicrobials. The antimicrobials should be administered within 24 h after exposure if possible and can consist of either a single dose of ceftriaxone 250 mg intramuscularly or ciprofloxacin 500 mg once in areas where ciprofloxacin resistance isolates of *Neisseria meningitidis* have not been detected. Rifampin dosed at 600 mg twice daily for 2 days is also effective as postexposure prophylaxis.

Polio Vaccine

The global polio vaccination initiative has led to a vast decrease in cases of polio. As of 2012, polio is endemic only in Afghanistan, Pakistan, and Nigeria with cases also being reported in Chad, Congo, and Angola. HCW can rarely be exposed to poliovirus in secretions from infected patients. The use of polio vaccination is recommended for HCW who may be at a higher risk of acquiring the disease if work in a laboratory handles specimens that may harbor polioviruses or HCW in areas of endemic polio [2]. The use of a single dose of the inactivated vaccine (IPV) is recommended for HCW who have had the primary polio vaccination. HCW who have not had the polio vaccination earlier should receive a three-dose series of IPV with the second dose 4–8 weeks after the first dose and the third dose 6–12 months after the second dose.

Other Vaccines

As adults HCW may be recommended other vaccines based on age as well as other individual risk factors such as the pneumococcal vaccination, tetanus and diphtheria toxoid (Td) based on age, or the presence of certain chronic medical problems. These and other vaccinations received by the HCW should be recorded in the HCW medical record. The health-care facilities should ensure that they have policies and procedures developed to ensure all HCW can achieve high vaccination rates of vaccine-preventable diseases. The vaccination medical records should be reviewed annually to ensure that newly hired HCW can also achieve high vaccination rates. This strategy can lead to the prevention of nosocomial outbreaks of vaccine-preventable diseases.

Summary

The optimum use of vaccines among HCW is an extremely valuable tool for infection prevention among HCW. The achievement of high rates of vaccination among HCW can lead to protection of HCW from serious complications from vaccine-preventable diseases and also prevent the HCW from acting as a vector for disseminating infections to patients especially immunocompromised patients who may not mount an adequate immunological response themselves to vaccines. Health-care facilities and infection preventionists should aim for high rates of vaccine uptake among all HCW.

References

1. Weber DJ, Weigle K, Rutala WA. Vaccines for healthcare workers. In: Plotkin SA, Orenstein WA, editors. Vaccines. 3rd ed. Philadelphia: WB Saunders Company; 1999.
2. Shefer A, Atkinson W, Friedman C, Kuhar DT, et al. Immunization of health-care personnel. MMWR Recomm Rep. 2011;60:1–45.
3. Bolyard EA, Tablan OC, Williams WW, et al. Guideline for infection control in healthcare personnel. Infect Control Hosp Epidemiol. 1998;19(6):407–63.
4. Miller BL, Ahmed F, Lindley MC, et al. Institutional requirements for influenza vaccination of healthcare personnel: results from a nationally representative survey of acute care hospitals—United States. Clin Infect Dis. 2011;53(11):1051–9.
5. Poland GA, Haiduven DJ. Immunization in the health care worker. In: APIC, editor. Text of infection control and epidemiology. Washington, DC: Association for Professionals in Infection Control and Epidemiology; 2002. p. 80.1–80.32.
6. Weber DJ, Rutala WA, Weigle K. Selection and use of vaccines for healthcare workers. Infect Control Hosp Epidemiol. 1997;18(10):682–7.
7. Mahoney FJ, Stewart K, Hu H, et al. Progress toward the elimination of hepatitis B virus transmission among health care workers in the United States. Arch Inter Med. 1997;157(22):2601.

8. Werner BG, Grady GF. Accidental hepatitis-B-surface-antigen-positive inoculations. Use of e antigen to estimate infectivity. Ann Intern Med. 1982;7(3):367.
9. Recommendations for preventing transmission of infections among chronic hemodialysis patients. MMWR. 2001;50(RR-5):1–63.
10. Dienstag JL, Werner BG, Polk BF, et al. Hepatitis B vaccine in health care personnel: safety, immunogenicity, and indicators of efficacy. Ann Intern Med. 1984;101(1):34.
11. Grady GF, Lee VA, Prince AM, et al. Hepatitis B immune globulin for accidental exposures among medical personnel: final report of a multicenter controlled trial. J Infect Dis. 1978;138(5):625–38.
12. Meyers JD, MacQuarrie MB, Merigan TC, et al. Nosocomial varicella: part I: outbreak in oncology patients at a children's hospital. West J Med. 1979;130(3):196.
13. Hyams PS, Stuewe M, Heitzer V. Herpes zoster causing varicella (chickenpox) in hospital employees: cost of a casual attitude. Am J Infect Control. 1984;12(1):2–5.
14. Yoshikawa T, Ihira M, Suzuki K, et al. Rapid contamination of the environments with varicella zoster virus DNA from a patient with herpes zoster. J Med Virol. 2001;63(1):64–6.
15. Haiduven-Griffiths D, Fecko H. Varicella in hospital personnel: a challenge for the infection control practitioner. Am J Infect Control. 1987;15(5):207–11.
16. Weber DJ, Rutala WA, Hamilton H. Prevention and control of varicella-zoster infections in healthcare facilities. Infect Control Hosp Epidemiol. 1996;17:694–705.
17. Chadha MS, Broor S, Gunasekaran P, et al. Multisite virological influenza surveillance in India: 2004–2008. Influenza Other Respir Viruses. 2011;6(3):196–203.
18. Saxen H, Virtanen M. Randomized, placebo-controlled double blind study on the efficacy of influenza immunization on absenteeism of health care workers. Pediatr Infect Dis J. 1999;18(9):779–83.
19. Potter J, Stott DJ, Roberts MA, et al. Influenza vaccination of health care workers in long-term-care hospitals reduces the mortality of elderly patients. J Infect Dis. 1997;175(1):1–6.
20. Hayward AC, Harling R, Wetten S, et al. Effectiveness of an influenza vaccine programme for care home staff to prevent death, morbidity, and health service use among residents: cluster randomized controlled trial. BMJ. 2006;333(7581):1241.
21. Babcock HM, Gemeinhart N, Jones M, et al. Mandatory influenza vaccination of health care workers: translating policy to practice. Clin Infect Dis. 2010;50(4):459–64.
22. C. D. C. Measles, mumps, and rubella–vaccine use and strategies for elimination of measles, rubella, and congenital rubella syndrome and control of mumps: recommendations of the Advisory Committee on Immunization Practices (ACIP). MMWR. 1998;47:1–57.
23. Chen SY, Anderson S, Kutty PK, et al. Health care–associated measles outbreak in the United States after an importation: challenges and economic impact. J Infect Dis. 2011;203(11):1517–25.
24. Steingart KR, Thomas AR, Dykewicz CA, et al. Transmission of measles virus in healthcare settings during a communitywide outbreak. Infect Control Hosp Epidemiol. 1999;20(2):115–19.
25. Deville JG, Cherry JD, Christenson PD, et al. Frequency of unrecognized Bordetella pertussis infections in adults. Clin Infect Dis. 1995;21(3):639–42.
26. Wright SW, Decker MD, Edwards KM. Incidence of pertussis infection in healthcare workers. Infect Control Hosp Epidemiol. 1999;20(2):120–3.
27. Calugar A, Ortega-Sánchez IR, Tiwari T, et al. Nosocomial pertussis: costs of an outbreak and benefits of vaccinating health care workers. Clin Infect Dis. 2006;42(7):981–8.
28. Chodick G, Ashkenazi S, Lerman Y. The risk of hepatitis A infection among healthcare workers: a review of reported outbreaks and sero-epidemiologic studies. J Hosp Infect. 2006;62(4):414–20.
29. Kak V, Sundareshan V, Modi J, et al. Immunotherapies in infectious diseases. Med Clin North Am. 2012;96(3):455.
30. Mermin JH, Townes JM, Gerber M, et al. Typhoid fever in the United States, 1985–1994: changing risks of international travel and increasing antimicrobial resistance. Arch Intern Med. 1998;158(6):633.
31. Sejvar JJ, Johnson D, Popovic T, et al. Assessing the risk of laboratory-acquired meningococcal disease. J Clin Microbiol. 2005;43(9):4811–14.

Part III

Current Practices for Infection Prevention in the Hospital Settings

Current Practices for Infection Prevention in the Hospital Settings

3

Alice Haynes and Nancy Khardori

Introduction

The principles and practices aimed at prevention and control of hospital-acquired infections are directed at various links in the chain of transmission. They include the following: (1) to contain or eliminate the reservoirs of agents and/or to curtail the persistence of agents in a specific setting, (2) to protect the host against disease caused by microorganisms, and (3) to interrupt the transmission of infection. Interventions to modify environmental reservoirs are aimed at interrupting the transmission for these inanimate environmental sources. The barriers, e.g., masks, were used to keep the smells and "contagion" away even before the germ theory of disease was conceived. The appropriate barriers now include gloves, gowns, and eye protection for blood/body fluid–borne infections and high-filtration masks for infections transmitted by droplet nuclei. The most important and effective nosocomial infection control intervention remains the routine washing of hands before, between, and

A. Haynes, RN, CIC
BonSecours DePaul Medical Center, Norfolk, VA, USA

N. Khardori, M.D., Ph.D. (✉)
Division of Infectious Diseases, Department of Internal Medicine, Eastern Virginia Medical School, Norfolk, VA, USA

Department of Microbiology and Molecular Cell Biology, Eastern Virginia Medical School, Norfolk, VA, USA
e-mail: nkhardori@gmail.com

after patient contact in healthcare settings. This chapter focuses on the interruption of transmission of infectious agents in the hospital setting by Standard Precautions recommended for all patients and "isolation" of patients using precautions based on known methods of transmission.

Historically, hospital construction before 1850 featured open wards where cross infection was common and mortality rates were high in urban hospitals [1]. Based on the observations during the Crimean war, Florence Nightingale advocated small pavilion – type wards joined by open-air corridors [2]. She also emphasized the importance of asepsis and a clean environment. The germ theory of disease was accepted in the US hospitals in late 1800s leading to decrease in overcrowding and increase in antisepsis. Individual and group isolation was used by "communicable disease" hospitals as early as 1989 [3]. General hospitals began to isolate patients with communicable diseases in individual rooms with the use of separate utensils and disinfectant by the turn of the century [4]. The theory of communicability by contact rather than airborne spread for most diseases was promoted in France [5]. This allowed patients with communicable diseases to be housed in general wards with separation by wire screens. In addition to separating the patient from others, the barrier served as a reminder for hospital staff to wear gowns and wash hands. This is how the trend of caring for patient with communicable disease in the general hospitals rather than isolation/fever hospitals started in the United States. In the early twentieth century, it was demonstrated that fumigation had no effect on the secondary cases emphasizing the role of persons rather than things as spreaders of disease [6, 7]. The concept of cohorting, allowing patients with communicable diseases to be housed in the same room as other patients, was first applied in the Providence City Hospital [5]. The barrier techniques needed for each patient were put on a card placed on the patient's bed. The development of infection control programs in the US hospitals was prompted by the emergence of Staphylococcus aureus as a hospital pathogen in the late 1950s. The first edition of American Hospital Association's manual in 1968 presented a simple barrier precautions scheme for patients with communicable diseases and listed the need for gloves, gowns, masks, and visitor screening [7]. The CDC, while conducting nosocomial outbreak investigations in the 1960s, recognized the need for standardized policies for isolating hospitalized patients with communicable diseases [8]. The first CDC isolation recommendations were published in 1970 [9]. This manual listed seven categories of isolation: strict isolation, respiratory isolation, enteric precautions, wound and skin precautions, discharge precautions, blood precautions, and protective isolation. Many of the practices described in the manual are applicable to any hospitalized patient. Application of poor techniques when handling uninfected patients can only result in sense of false security. Updates to the CDC manual were made in 1975and 1978. In 1983, substantial changes were made to the recommendations including the use of the word "guidelines." The CDC series Guidelines for the Prevention and Control of Nosocomial Infections that has followed is now the state of the art in infection control practices. These guidelines have accepted and customized for medical management of bioterrorism threats [10].

Standard Precautions

In 1985, the Centers for Disease Control and Prevention (CDC) introduced Universal Precautions (UP) to hospitals for the protection of healthcare personnel as a response to the emergence of HIV/AIDS. Another initiative, Body Substance Isolation, soon followed. The CDC recognized there was confusion created by Universal Precautions and Body Substance Isolation, so in 1996, they published new guidelines with a two-tiered method, Standard Precautions and Transmission-based Precautions. The CDC, in cooperation with the Healthcare Infection Control Practices Advisory Committee (HICPAC), established Standard Precautions to address the prevention of the spread of infectious agents in healthcare settings and are the result of combining the key components from Universal Precautions and Body Substance Isolation along with the understanding that all blood and body fluids, except sweat, are potentially infectious, and inanimate objects are potentially contaminated with infectious agents, therefore are capable of being reservoirs in the chain of transmission of infectious agents [11, 12]. Does the term, "Standard," downplay the role and significance of these precautions? Absolutely not, the message is that this is the expected way to prevent the spread of disease and applies to every encounter between patients and healthcare providers.

Standard Precautions group together infection prevention practices consisting of the use of Personal Protective Equipment (PPE), such as gowns, gloves, masks, goggles or face shields, and the performance of hand hygiene, washing hands with soap and water, especially when they are visibly soiled, or using an alcohol-based hand sanitizer. The basic premise for these practices is the need to anticipate a potential source of exposure, and take precautions by donning the appropriate barrier that will provide protection. For example, gloves should be worn when contact with blood, body fluid, or contaminated surfaces are likely. When the risk of being splashed by a potentially infectious substance exists, a mask and eye protection should be worn. A gown may be worn to protect clothing as well. Care should be taken when handling soiled linen and patient care equipment to reduce contamination of the environment with infectious agents.

Standard Precautions have been found to be an effective means of preventing the transmission of infectious agents in all healthcare settings. The Centers for Disease Control and Prevention recommend that Standard Precautions be implemented for all patient encounters, whether the risk of transmitting an infectious agent is suspected or has been confirmed; all patients are to be thought of as potentially able to transmit.

Another component of Standard Precautions is the potential contamination of items in the patient's environment and appropriate measures to reduce the risk from inanimate sources. When handling or having direct contact with patient care equipment or other items in a patient's environment that potentially have been exposed to infectious agents, gloves should be worn followed by performing hand hygiene after removing gloves. When it is not practical to dedicate equipment to individual patients, proper cleaning and disinfecting or sterilizing is recommended before use on another patient.

Standard Precautions were originally established to protect healthcare personnel by reducing their risk of exposure to infectious agents. But in recent years, the importance of the protection of the patient has been recognized. The need for changes and reinforcement of proper infection control practices, as part of the practice of Standard Precautions, was identified as the result of outbreak investigations. From those investigations came the recommendations for Respiratory Etiquette/Cough Etiquette, Safe Injection Practices, and donning a mask during lumbar puncture procedures.

Respiratory Etiquette/Cough Etiquette is a practice that was implemented to reduce the spread of respiratory illnesses. During the SARS outbreak in 2003, emergency departments needed a way to control transmission of the disease, and putting a mask on a patient who has symptoms of a respiratory illness such as cough, increased production of respiratory secretions, and fever at the first stage of encounter in a healthcare facility has been shown to be effective. Healthcare facilities are expected to have masks, tissues, a waste receptacle, and hand hygiene products available with signage to explain their use at points of entry into the facility and in waiting areas.

Patients should be taught to use a tissue to cover their cough or sneeze, discard the tissue in a wastebasket, and wash their hands to reduce the risk of spreading infection.

The need to address injection practices was recognized in response to hepatitis B and C outbreak investigations that were caused by the use of poor technique during the administration of medications by injection. Used needles reinserted into a multidose vial or bag of saline and administration of intravenous injections to multiple patients using a single needle/syringe were two of the major breaks in infection control practices that were found to have led to the outbreaks. The need to educate healthcare personnel resulted in the establishment of "The One & Only Campaign," meaning one needle, one syringe, and only one time use for one patient. Safe Injection Practices dictate that used needles never be recapped, removed from disposable syringes, bent, broken or manipulated by hand, and are disposed of in puncture-resistant containers to prevent sharps injuries.

Wearing a mask to protect the patient has become a part of performing a lumbar puncture procedure after several patients were found to have acquired meningitis following a myelogram.

The expectation is that a mask will be worn whenever a catheter in placed or an injection administered into the spinal or epidural space.

Transmission-Based Precautions

In addition to Standard Precautions, Transmission-based Precautions are implemented when more restrictive measures are needed to decrease the risk of the spread of infection. The precautions taken to contain the known or suspected infectious agents are determined by their mode of transmission. A patient suspected of having, known to have, or in the case of Multidrug-Resistant Organisms, when a patient has a history of infection or colonization and there is a risk of transmission to others, the need to isolate the patient is important for the protection of others. There are three types of Transmission-based Precautions: Contact, Droplet, and Airborne. Contact Precautions are implemented when acquisition of a pathogen can occur by touching or coming in direct contact with a patient or the articles in the patient's environment. Illnesses spread by respiratory droplets are prevented from transmission by Droplet Precautions. These infectious agents can be spread by being expelled in respiratory secretions during coughing, sneezing, or talking, but because the particles are large, they drop to the ground within 3–6 ft of the patient and do not pose a threat for those at a greater distance. There are some respiratory illnesses that require Airborne Precautions. Airborne Precautions require a room with special air handling capability. Negative pressure is established in the room, so that the particles, known to remain floating in the air for extended periods of time, can be ventilated to the outside or forced through an HEPA filtration system before the air is returned to circulate in the facility.

Contact Precautions, in Addition to Standard Precautions

Contact Precautions require that a gown and gloves be worn to protect the healthcare worker while performing patient care activities. It is recommended that the gown and gloves be put on prior to entering the room. This combination of PPE can also impact the safety of other patients that are being cared for by the same healthcare worker and may potentially be exposed to pathogens that can be transported to them on the caregiver's clothing. Hand hygiene is a key component of Contact Precautions. Hands should be washed with soap and water, or an alcohol-based hand sanitizer product used, prior to putting PPE on and after removing it.

Examples of Illnesses Requiring Contact Precautions

- When patient is known or suspected to have an illness transmitted by direct contact with the patient or by contact with articles in the patient's environment

All Multidrug-Resistant Organisms

Gastrointestinal, respiratory, skin, or wound infections or colonization with multidrug-resistant bacteria judged by the infection control program, based on current state, regional, or national recommendations, to be of special clinical and epidemiologic significance

Enteric infections with a low infectious dose or prolonged environmental survival, including:

For diapered or incontinent patients: enterohemorrhagic *Escherichia coli* O157:H7, *Shigella*, hepatitis A, or rotavirus

Respiratory syncytial virus, parainfluenza virus, or enteroviral infections in infants and young children

Skin infections that are highly contagious or that may occur on dry skin, including:

Diphtheria (cutaneous)

Herpes simplex virus (neonatal or disseminated)

Impetigo

Major (noncontained) abscesses, cellulitis, or decubiti

Pediculosis

Scabies

Staphylococcal furunculosis in infants and young children

Zoster (disseminated or in the immunocompromised host)†

Viral/hemorrhagic conjunctivitis

Viral hemorrhagic infections (Ebola, Lassa, or Marburg)

Interventions Used When Implementing Contact Precautions

- Patient and visitor education.
- Signage for patient's room.
- Availability of PPE (gowns and gloves).
- Gown and gloves worn on entry to room.
- Use dedicated or disposable equipment.
- Upon exiting, PPE is discarded inside the room.
- Hand hygiene: Hand washing with soap and water or an alcohol-based hand sanitizer.
- Limit transport of patient.
- Clean room daily, focusing on frequently touched surfaces.

Special Contact Precautions, in Addition to Standard Precautions

Special Contact Precautions may be necessary for patients infected with a spore-forming organism. ***Clostridium difficile infection*** (CDI),

Norovirus, or any organism that is resistant to the usual hospital cleaners and disinfectants require different means to reduce the risk of transmission of disease.

Interventions Used When Implementing Special Contact Precautions

- Hand washing with soap and water before and after contact with the patient, scrubbing to create slight friction to mechanically mobilize any organism that may be on the hands, and rinsing well to flush the organism off the skin.
- Meticulous cleaning of room with an EPA-approved, hospital grade cleaner, followed by disinfecting with a 1:10 bleach solution, especially frequently touched surfaces.
- Use dedicated or disposable equipment.

Respiratory or Droplet Precautions, in Addition to Standard Precautions

Droplet Precautions should be implemented when caring for a patient with a respiratory infection or when there is risk of exposure to respiratory secretions or contact with mucous membranes. Placing the patient in a private room is preferred, but when a single-patient room is not available, an assessment of risk to other patients should be done before placing an infectious patient with others. If it is necessary to place multiple patients in the same room, separating them by three or more feet and having a privacy curtain drawn between them is important. Teaching patients to practice Respiratory Etiquette can also help reduce the transmission of infectious agents.

Interventions Used When Implementing Droplet Precautions

- Hand hygiene.
- Private room preferred, but not required; patients with the same disease can be placed in the same room.
- Surgical/procedural mask is worn by care providers and put on before entering the room.

- Handle items contaminated with respiratory secretions with gloves.
- Use dedicated or disposable equipment.
- Upon exiting, PPE is discarded inside the room.
- Clean room daily, focusing on frequently touched surfaces.
- Patient should only leave room for essential test, and wear a surgical/procedural mask when out of their room.

Examples of Illnesses Requiring Droplet Precautions
- When patient is known or suspected to have an illnesses transmitted by large particle droplets
 Invasive *Haemophilus influenzae* type b disease, including meningitis, pneumonia, epiglottitis, and sepsis
 Invasive *Neisseria meningitidis* disease, including meningitis, pneumonia, and sepsis
 Other serious bacterial respiratory infections spread by droplet transmission, including:
 Diphtheria (pharyngeal)
 Mycoplasma pneumonia
 Pertussis
 Pneumonic plague
 Streptococcal (group A) pharyngitis, pneumonia, or scarlet fever in infants and young children
 Serious viral infections spread by droplet transmission, including:
 Adenovirus
 Influenza
 Mumps Parvovirus B19
 Rubella

Airborne Precautions, in Addition to Standard Precautions

A patient requiring Airborne Isolation Precautions should be placed in a room capable of supporting negative pressure airflow. The air should be vented outside or filtered before being circulated in the facility. The air pressure in the room should be tested daily while it is occupied with a confirmed or suspected infectious patient. All healthcare providers wear an N-95 respirator on entry to the room. If a room capable of providing negative pressure is not available, the patient may be placed in a single-patient room and wear a surgical/procedural mask as tolerated, until an Airborne Illness Isolation Room is available.

Interventions Used When Implementing Airborne Precautions

- Hand hygiene.
- Patient is placed in an Airborne Illness Isolation Room (AIIR)/Negative Pressure.
- Door remains closed.
- Limit transport of patient for essential tests only, and when necessary patient wears a surgical/procedural mask outside their room.
- Use dedicated or disposable equipment.
- Fit-tested N-95 level respirator is put on before entering room.
- Respirator is removed only after exiting room with the door closed.
  Examples of Illnesses Requiring Airborne Precautions
- When a patient is known, or suspected, to have an illness transmitted by airborne droplet nuclei that can be suspended in the air and remains infectious for long distances
  Measles
  Varicella (including disseminated zoster)
  Tuberculosis

Strict Isolation

Strict Isolation was introduced in 1970 as one of the seven categories of isolation precautions. It continued to be included as a category through the 1983 revision when the precautions became more disease-specific and was practiced until the guideline for Universal Precautions was published. Isolation practices at that time were simple and required little decision making by the healthcare team members. The isolation category for patients with infections transmissible by more than one route is a combination of above-described categories, e.g., a combination of contact and airborne precautions for varicella.

Quarantine

The practice of quarantine is used to prevent the potential spread of disease when it is suspected that a person who is currently well may have been exposed to a communicable disease. By law, a person can be held, separated from others, or confined to their home to wait out an illness's incubation period to determine if they become ill [13].

Examples of communicable diseases that are Quarantinable:
Cholera
Diphtheria
Infectious tuberculosis
Plague
Smallpox
Yellow fever
Viral hemorrhagic fevers
SARS
New types of influenza that have the potential to cause a pandemic

Summary

It is obvious that for a hospital to just say that they have and follow the CDC guidelines for prevention of transmission of infectious agents is rather bureaucratic and simplistic. The actual implementation is absolutely dependent on behavioral changes needed to support improvements in the areas of personal hygiene, specifically in the washing of hands between tasks in preparation of food, caring for children, and caring for the sick in the hospital and non-hospital settings. In the hospital setting, risks of transmission to other patients especially those with serious comorbidities and immunocompromising conditions are associated with morbidity, mortality, and cost. It is not uncommon to see healthcare workers using personal protective equipment inappropriately. For example, if a gown is not worn and tied properly, it actually be falling on top of the patient and other surfaces and become more likely to pick and transmit microorganisms. If it is not disposed properly, flows out of containers, the organisms can be aerosolized and transmitted in more than one way. It is the responsibility of everyone not just a few infection preventionists in the hospital to understand the principles and implement the practices of infection prevention. The practices the healthcare providers believe which protect them and their families are more likely to be adhered to. In this regard, the significance of basic hand hygiene principles seems to be least valued and understood. On the other hand, they can be overzealous about isolation precautions in a given patient based on profiling and misconceptions leading to their isolation from care. Unfortunately, this collateral damage has not received much attention. It is fair to say that as healthcare providers of all types, we have not reached a balanced and fully understood level in infection prevention practices 45 years after they were first formalized. One of the major reasons is the fact that during formative medical school years, the teaching of basic and applied sciences like microbiology is de-emphasized, and getting into the glamorous realm of clinical medicine very early is encouraged at the cost of learning fundamentals.

Resource constrained settings cannot justify to deviate from the guidelines necessary to prevent HAI. The abovementioned measures have been spelled out in simple language to help implementation in letter and spirit.

References

1. Bordley J, Harvey AM. Two centuries of American medicine, 1776–1976. Philadelphia: W.B. Saunders; 1976.
2. Richardson DL. Aseptic fever nursing. Am J Nurs. 1915;15:1082–93.
3. Aronson SP. Communicable disease nursing. Garden City: Medical Examination Publishing; 1978.
4. Chapin CV. The sources and modes of infection. 2nd ed. New York: Wiley; 1912.
5. Morrison ST, Arnold CR, editors. Communicable diseases by Landon and Sider. 9th ed. Philadelphia: F.A. Davis; 1969.
6. Anderson GW, Arnstein MG. Ancient concepts of transmission. Communicable disease control. 3rd ed. New York: Macmillan; 1953.
7. American Hospital Association. Infection control in the hospital. Chicago: American Hospital Association; 1968.
8. Garner JS, Hughes JM. Options for isolation precautions. Ann Intern Med. 1987;107:248–50.
9. Centers for Disease Control. Isolation techniques for use in hospitals. DHEW publication no. (PHS)*70-2054. Washington, DC: U.S. Government Printing Office. 1970.
10. United States Army Medical Institute of Infectious Diseases. Medical management of biological casualties handbook, 7th ed. 2011. Available at http://www.usamriid.army.mil/education/bluebookpdf/USAMRIID
11. APIC textbook of infection control and epidemiology, 3rd ed. 2009.
12. Siegel J, Rhinehart E, Jackson M, et al., and the Healthcare Infection Control Practices Advisory Committee (HICPAC). Guideline for isolation precautions: preventing transmission of infectious agents in healthcare settings. 2007. Available at: http://www.cdc.gov/ncidod/dhqp/pdf/guidelines/Isolation2007.pdf
13. Centers for Disease Control and Prevention. About quarantine and isolation. Available at http://www.cdc.gov/quarantine

Part IV

Hospital Infection Prevention Program

Hospital Infection Prevention Program

4

Pallab Ray and Lipika Singhal

Introduction

Health care saves lives and has brought unprecedented benefits to generations of patients and their families. However, it also carries risks. Healthcare-associated infection (HAI) is sometimes the unfortunate consequence of modern medicine: new diagnostic and therapeutic procedures, new treatments for advanced malignancy, organ transplantation, and intensive care are associated with an increased risk of infection [1, 2].

HAI is also referred to as nosocomial infections that affect patients in a hospital or other healthcare facility and are not present or incubating at the time of admission. They also include infections acquired by patients in the hospital or healthcare facility but clinically manifest after discharge and occupational infections among staff. Escalating medical care costs have resulted in shorter hospital stays and higher volumes of outpatient surgical procedures. It is estimated that from 20 % to 70 % of postoperative surgical site infections do not become apparent until after the patient's discharge [3–5].

At any time, over 1.4 million people worldwide are suffering from infections acquired in the hospital. In the developed world, about 5–10 % of patients admitted to hospitals acquire one or more infections, whereas the risk of HAI in developing countries is 2–20 times higher than in developed countries; in some countries, the proportion can exceed 25 % [1, 6]. Some determinants which may contribute to higher HAI in developing countries are as follows:

- Inadequate environmental hygienic conditions and waste disposal
- Poor infrastructure
- Insufficient equipment
- Understaffing
- Overcrowding
- Poor knowledge and application of basic infection control measures
- Lack of proper procedure
- Lack of knowledge of injection and blood transfusion safety
- Absence of local and national guidelines and policies

HAI results in prolonged hospital stays, long-term disability, increased resistance of microorganisms to antimicrobials, and massive additional costs for patients, their families, and health systems and causes preventable deaths. A review found a minimum reduction effect of 10 % to a maximum of 70 %, depending on the setting, study design, baseline infection rates, and type of infection [6, 7].

Infection Control Committee

In the 1940s and 1950s, severe *Staphylococcus aureus* pandemics caused substantial morbidity and mortality in US hospitals. In part because of these pandemics, the Joint Commission on

P. Ray (✉) • L. Singhal
Department of Medical Microbiology, PGIMER,
Chandigarh, India
e-mail: drpallabray@gmail.com

Accreditation of Healthcare Organizations (JCAHO) in 1958 first recommended that hospitals should appoint infection control committees (ICC) with the primary role to reduce the risk of HAI, thereby protecting patients, healthcare personnel, and visitors [8]. Over the next 50 years, the field of infection control developed incrementally in response to medical advances by incorporating the science of epidemiology to elucidate risk factors for HAIs, so that interventions to prevent them could be tested and implemented.

However, there is a gap between the patient safety improvements that are currently possible and the improvements that are actually being made. This gap arises because existing tools and interventions are not being widely implemented.

An ICC provides a forum for multidisciplinary input and cooperation and information sharing. This committee should include wide representation from relevant programs, e.g., management, physicians, clinical microbiology, other healthcare workers, pharmacy, central supply, maintenance, housekeeping, and training services [9]. The optimal structure of ICC varies with the type, needs, and resources of the facility. Large hospitals with a high proportion of tertiary care patients require a more complex system to meet their needs. The ideal characteristics of committee members include the following: (1) an interest and commitment in infection control, (2) representation of a large multidisciplinary group within the hospital, (3) authority in their given specialty, (4) tact, and (5) charisma.

The goal of this interdisciplinary team is to bring together individuals with expertise in different areas of health care. The role of the ICC is multifaceted. It should be involved in planning, monitoring, evaluating, updating, and educating. The committee must have a reporting relationship directly to either administration or the medical staff to promote program visibility and effectiveness. In an emergency (such as an outbreak), this committee must be able to meet promptly [9].

Infection Prevention Coordinators

There has been an increasing focus on prevention over control of HAI. Individuals working in infection control have seen their titles change from infection control practitioner to infection control professional and most recently to infection preventionist (IP), emphasizing their critical role in protecting patients. They are expected not only to monitor infection rates but also to intervene, implement, and/or lead healthcare personnel in the implementation of processes aimed at reducing rates of infections [10, 11].

Over the past few decades, controlling HAIs has become highly technical. Therefore, the bulk of the ICC's work is best accomplished by a core of experts that includes the hospital epidemiologist, infection control professionals, a medical microbiologist, and the director of employee health. Policy formulations should be developed by this subgroup and, after thoughtful consideration, brought to the entire committee for review, ratification, and support from political and administrative standpoints.

The Role of the Key Infection Prevention Coordinators as Outlined by the World Health Organization

Role of Hospital Management

The administration and/or medical management of the hospital must provide leadership by supporting the hospital infection program [7]. They are responsible for the following:

- Establishing a multidisciplinary ICC
- Identifying appropriate resources for a program
- Monitoring infections and applying the most appropriate methods for preventing infection
- Ensuring education and training of all staff through support of programs on the prevention of infection, disinfection, and sterilization techniques
- Delegating technical aspects of hospital hygiene to appropriate staff, such as nursing and housekeeping
- Periodically reviewing the status of nosocomial infections and effectiveness of interventions to contain them
- Reviewing, approving, and implementing policies approved by the ICC

- Ensuring that the infection control team has authority to facilitate appropriate programs
- Participating in outbreak investigation

Role of Hospital Epidemiologist/ Physician

The hospital epidemiologist occupies a unique position. He directly supervises the infection control program and interacts with many hospital departments and specialities, hospital administrators, and extramural agencies. The position is generally held by a physician who is trained in infectious diseases with additional training in the discipline of epidemiology.

Specifically, physicians are responsible for the following:
- Protecting their own patients from other infected patients and from hospital staff who may be infected [12]
- Complying with the practices approved by the ICC
- Obtaining appropriate microbiological specimens when an infection is present or suspected
- Notifying cases of HAI to the team
- Complying with the recommendations of the Antimicrobial Use Committee regarding the use of antibiotics and advising patients, visitors, and staff on techniques to prevent the transmission of infection
- Instituting appropriate treatment for any infections they themselves have and taking steps to prevent such infections being transmitted to other individuals, especially patients

Role of the Medical Microbiologist

The clinical microbiology laboratory should be intimately involved in all aspects of the infection control program. At least one microbiologist should be a member of the ICC and act as a consultant to the infection control program. The laboratory, which is the source of microbiologic culture information, must provide easy access to high-quality, relevant, and timely data, and the microbiologist should give guidance and support on how to use the laboratory resources for epidemiologic

purposes. The microbiologist can link diagnosis and patient care within the institution to community healthcare issues that impact public health. This linkage provides the strength required to implement strategies that promote patient safety and healthcare quality. The microbiologists need to demonstrate leadership in this regard and work hard to carve a role for themselves as experts and facilitators in the process making the management and clinical teams to own up responsibility [13].

The microbiologist is responsible for the following:
- Handling patient and staff specimens to maximize the likelihood of a microbiological diagnosis
- Developing guidelines for appropriate collection, transport, and handling of specimens ensuring laboratory practices meet appropriate standards
- Ensuring safe laboratory practice to prevent infections in staff
- Performing antimicrobial susceptibility testing following internationally recognized methods and providing summary reports of prevalence of resistance
- Monitoring sterilization, disinfection, and the environment where necessary
- Timely communication of results to the ICC
- Epidemiological typing of hospital microorganisms where necessary

Role of the Nursing Staff

Implementation of patient care practices for ICP is the role of the nursing staff. Nurses should be professionally trained and familiar with such practices and maintain the same for all patients throughout the duration of their hospital stay.

The nurse in charge of infection control is a member of the infection control team and is responsible for the following:
- Identifying nosocomial infections
- Investigation of the type of infection and infecting organism
- Participating in training of personnel for surveillance of hospital infections
- Participating in outbreak investigation

- Development of infection control policy and review and approval of patient care policies relevant to infection control
- Ensuring compliance with local and national regulations in liaison with public health and other facilities where appropriate
- Providing expert consultative advice to staff health and other appropriate hospital programs in matters relating to transmission of infections
- Supervising the implementation of techniques for the prevention of infections in specialized areas such as the operating suite, the intensive care, maternity and newborn units besides monitoring of nursing adherence to policies

Role of the Central Sterilization Service

A central sterilization department serves all hospital areas, including the operating suite. An appropriately qualified individual must be responsible for management of the program. Responsibility for day-to-day management may be delegated to a nurse or other individual with appropriate qualifications, experience, and knowledge of medical devices.

The responsibilities of the central sterilization service are as follows:

- To clean, decontaminate, test, prepare for use, sterilize, and store aseptically all sterile hospital equipment
- To work in collaboration with the ICC and other hospital program to develop and monitor policies on cleaning and decontamination of reusable equipment, contaminated equipment including wrapping procedures

The purpose of the ICC is not to reduce the individual responsibility that each healthcare provider has, but to provide leadership for all employees throughout the facility. Many IPC measures such as hand hygiene and the correct application of basic precautions during invasive procedures are simple and low-cost, but require staff accountability and behavioral change. Close cooperation between the ICC and healthcare staff is essential in formulating and implementing

measures to avoid staff contracting or spreading infections in the course of their employment.

ICC is recommended to meet at least quarterly and should produce minutes of their meetings and produce an annual report. The ICC continues to acquire new skills and insight as they continue to confront practical problems on the ground. The management must ensure that the efforts to combat HAIs are supported by the management and made a core standard to be achieved.

The ICC has the following tasks [7]:

- To review and approve a yearly program of activity for surveillance and prevention.
- To review epidemiological surveillance data and identify areas for intervention.
- To assess and promote improved practice at all levels of the health facility.
- To ensure appropriate staff training in infection control and safety.
- To review risks associated with new technologies and monitor infectious risks of new devices and products, prior to their approval for use.
- To review and provide input into investigation of outbreaks.
- To communicate and cooperate with other committees of the hospital with common interests such as Pharmacy and Therapeutics or Antimicrobial Use Committee, Biosafety or Health and Safety Committees, and Blood Transfusion Committee.
- To standardize infection control procedures throughout the facility so that the same level of care is provided in all departments.
- The multidisciplinary composition of the committee makes it an ideal place to examine new product and procedure proposals from several aspects.

Surveillance

The word "surveillance" literally means "to watch over with great attention, authority, and often with suspicion." Surveillance is defined as "the ongoing, systematic collection, analysis, and interpretation of health data essential to the planning, implementation, and evaluation of public health practice, closely integrated with the timely dissemination of these data to those who need to know" [8].

The HAI rate in patients in a facility is an indicator of quality and safety of care. Through the infection surveillance system, the infection control program collects data on nosocomial infections in the hospital, the pathogens and their patterns of antimicrobial resistance, the factors that contributed to the infections, and their outcomes, ultimately aiming to reduce the nosocomial infections and their costs [7].

An effective surveillance is essential to determine the endemic rates of infection. Once these rates have been established, an outbreak can be identified when its rate of occurrence is significantly higher than the endemic rate [13].

The scientific value of surveillance was demonstrated by the 1985 landmark Study on the Efficacy of Nosocomial Infection Control (SENIC) [14]. This study validated the cost-benefit of infection control and indicated that a highly efficient active surveillance and infection control system could reduce the HAI rates by one-third (32 %). It also demonstrated that, to be effective, infection prevention programs must include (1) organized surveillance and control activities, (2) adequate number of trained infection control staff, and (3) a system for reporting SSI rates to surgeons [14].

A hospital should have clear goals for doing surveillance. Furthermore, these goals must be reviewed and updated frequently to meet new infection risks in changing patient populations, the introduction of new high-risk medical interventions, and changing pathogens and their resistance to antibiotics [8].

A valid surveillance system constitutes the backbone of infection prevention and control. There are several models of surveillance for HAI in different settings but all include the following:
1. The patients and units to be monitored (defined population)
2. A standardized set of case definitions and relevant information to be collected for each case
3. A method for detecting infections (numerators)

4. A method for detecting the exposed population (denominators)
5. The process for the analysis of data and calculation of rates
6. Methods for calculation

The specific objectives of a surveillance program include [1, 7] *the following*:
- To improve awareness of clinical staff and other hospital workers (including administrators) about nosocomial infections and antimicrobial resistance, so they appreciate the need for preventive action
- To monitor trends: incidence and distribution of nosocomial infections, prevalence, and, where possible, risk-adjusted incidence for intra- and inter-hospital comparisons
- To identify the need for new or intensified prevention programs and evaluate the impact of prevention measures
- To identify possible areas for improvement in patient care and for further epidemiological studies (i.e., risk factor analysis) at the hospital level

Key points in the process of surveillance for nosocomial infection rates are [7] *as follows*:
- Active surveillance (prevalence and incidence studies)
- Targeted surveillance (site-, unit-, priority-oriented)
- Appropriately trained investigators
- Standardized methodology
- Risk-adjusted rates for comparisons

Active surveillance (prevalence or incidence study) is recommended and must be done actively and frequently or even on daily basis, seeking out HAI, reporting them and implementing control measures for each case.

Prevalence Study (Cross Sectional/Transverse)

Infections in all patients hospitalized (hospital-wide surveillance) at a given point in time are identified (point prevalence) in the entire hospital or on selected units. Hospital-wide surveillance activities are highly time consuming, beyond the ability of most hospitals, and need to be balanced with the time needed for prevention and control activities. Typically, a team of trained investigators visits every patient of the hospital on a single day, reviewing medical and nursing charts, interviewing the clinical staff to identify infected patients, and collecting risk factor data.

The outcome measure is a prevalence rate. Prevalence rates are influenced by duration of the patient's stay and duration of infections. Another problem is determining whether an infection is still "active" on the day of the study. In spite of these limitations, hospital-wide surveillance increases awareness of nosocomial infection problems among clinical staff and increases the visibility of the infection control team. It is useful when initiating a surveillance program to assess current issues for all units, for all kinds of infections, and in all patients, before proceeding to a more focused continuing active surveillance program.

Incidence Study (Continuous/ Longitudinal)

Prospective identification of new infections (incidence surveillance) requires monitoring of all patients within a defined population for a specified time period. Patients are followed throughout their stay and sometimes after discharge (e.g., post-discharge surveillance for surgical site infections). This type of *Targeted Outcome surveillance* provides attack rates, infection ratio, and incidence rates. Tracking infection rates is necessary to compare the hospital's infection experience with that at other hospitals or at its own hospital over time. To make valid comparisons, the infection rates must be adjusted for the most important intrinsic and extrinsic risks of infection. When risk-adjusted infection rates are compared, significant variations in the rates may suggest the need for further investigation to identify possible infection control problems.

Recent trends in *Targeted Surveillance* include the following:

1. *Site-oriented surveillance*: Priorities will be to monitor frequent infections with significant impact in mortality, morbidity, and costs and which may be avoidable. This surveillance is primarily laboratory-based. The infection control program must have access to all patient and hospital records. The laboratory also provides units with regular reports on distribution of microorganisms isolated and antibiotic susceptibility profiles for the most frequent pathogens.

Common priority areas include the following:
- Ventilator-associated pneumonia (a high mortality rate)
- Surgical site infections (first for extrahospital days and cost)
- Primary (intravascular line) bloodstream infections (high mortality)
- Multiple drug-resistant bacteria

The ICC should set practical aims, for example, to reduce the incidence of surgical site infections (SSI) by a defined percentage in a defined period in the general surgical wards or to reduce the incidence of central venous access device infections by a defined percentage in a defined period in the intensive care unit. This strategy saves considerable resources. Once the capacity is established, a system of basic surveillance to identify any outbreak of HAIs can be incorporated to this surveillance strategy [13].

2. *Unit-oriented surveillance*: This surveillance targets areas of the hospital where the highest rates of infection, highest impact of infection, and antibiotic resistance are likely to be found. These areas include ICUs, cardiothoracic surgery units, and hematology and oncology units.

3. *Priority-oriented surveillance*: Surveillance undertaken for a specific issue of concern to the facility (i.e., urinary tract infections in patients with urinary catheters in long-term care facilities).

The highest quality surveillance methodology for HAIs was developed by the Centers for Disease Control and Prevention (CDC) and is unit based, infection site specific, and risk adjusted (i.e., expressed in terms of device-specific denominators).

Process Surveillance (or Clinical Audit): The aim of process surveillance or clinical audit is to observe/monitor compliance to the infection control practices against a set standard by the clinical staff. This process is continued with remedial measures instituted in real time as and when necessary until the practice meets the recommended standard [15].

In India, the National Communicable Diseases Centre (NCDC) is the principal laboratory division that is technically and administratively responsible for the entire nation's health service laboratories for communicable disease surveillance.

Nosocomial Outbreak Investigation

An outbreak is defined as an unusual or unexpected increase of a particular disease as compared to the background rate. It occurs in a particular time frame (brief interval), involves a specific patient population with well-defined susceptibility factors, and is caused by a single microbial strain from a point source or index case [7].

Often, outbreaks are associated with specific communicable diseases or specific procedures or devices used in hospital settings. Transmission of respiratory infections, viral gastroenteritis, or multidrug-resistant organisms like vancomycin-resistant enterococci (VRE), carbapenem-resistant *Acinetobacter baumannii* (CRAB), and *Clostridium difficile* are few examples of infections in the hospital setting [16, 17].

A timely and appropriate investigation is required to identify the source and vehicle of the outbreak and to implement most appropriate measures to control it and prevent further recurrences. This can sometimes lead to identification of new agents, reservoirs, or modes of transmission. This is also important in terms of morbidity, costs, and institutional image [18].

Essential steps in the management of an outbreak in hospital setting are [7, 8] as follows:

1. *Recognition of an outbreak.*
   - Data accumulated by ongoing surveillance allow detection of nosocomial outbreaks when they reveal an increase in reported cases or an unusual clustering of cases by time and place.
     - As epidemiologic investigation requires a retrospective review of data, laboratory records should be retained for at least 2 years in a readily accessible format like a logbook. This permits an analysis of long-term trends by providing baseline and a seasonally adjusted control.
   - An astute observation of a potential cluster of infections (at least two or more laboratory-confirmed cases) by physicians, nurses, or the microbiologist may also warrant investigation.
     - In the early stages of an outbreak, the causative agent may not be known; hence, an outbreak may also be suspected based on the presenting symptoms.
   - An investigation is definitely warranted under the following circumstances:
     - When the number of affected (or exposed) persons is large
     - When the disease is rare or severe
     - When there occurs a microbial or chemical contamination of food or water (infectious incidents)
     - When the outbreak has the potential to affect others unless prompt control measures are taken

2. *Notification of a suspected outbreak of infection.*
   - Any suspicion of an outbreak should be vigilantly notified to the appropriate individuals and departments in the institution.
   - An outbreak team is constituted with Infection Control Staff being a part of the outbreak team.

3. *Steps for investigating an outbreak* [7, 8].
   - Verify the diagnosis using clinical, epidemiological, and laboratory test information, considering seasonal disease occurrence.
   - Develop a working case definition based on clinical and laboratory criteria. The inclusion and exclusion criteria for cases must be precisely identified. A gradient of definition (as definite, probable or possible case) is often helpful. The definition should also differentiate between infection and colonization.

- The clinical diagnosis will usually be confirmed microbiologically. Optimal diagnostic specimens should be collected for microbiological investigations and sent to laboratory with clinical details.
- Consultant Medical Microbiologist should identify and perform antimicrobial susceptibility for all the clinical isolates obtained and should preserve them for further analysis.
- Using the case definition, evaluate statistically whether the current rates are significantly higher than pre-outbreak rates.
- Find cases systematically and plot an *epidemic curve* which is a graphic representation of the distribution of cases by time of onset.
  - Epidemic curve helps to distinguish between definite and probable cases.
  - The shape of the epidemic curve may suggest a single point source, ongoing transmission, or an intermittent source.
- Review the charts of case patients, and develop line lists containing demographic data (dates of admission and procedures, ward locations, dates) and exposure to potential risk factors.
  - Plot a time line with data for all common events. The number of cases is plotted on the y-axis, and the time interval between infection and potential risk factor (e.g., procedure, medication, contact with potentially infected patient or healthcare worker) is plotted on the x-axis.
- Review the literature about risk factors and potential sources, and compare them with those obtained in the present problem.
- Reinstitute standard hygiene precautions and infection control measures. Reemphasize hand hygiene among residents, staff, and visitors. The Centers for Disease Control and Prevention (CDC) has identified hand washing as the single most important means of preventing the spread of infection at all times [12].
- If it is found that no outbreak exists, concerned healthcare staff should be reassured,

and care taken to ensure that they are not discouraged from further reporting in the future.

4. *If outbreak exists, formulate a hypothesis regarding the source of infection and the probable mechanism of transmission.*
   - *Establish the source of infection*: Conduct environmental investigation by obtaining cultures of suspected common sources including testing of food and environmental samples where appropriate [8].
     - Clinical microbiology laboratory should perform environmental cultures to assess microbial contamination of inanimate objects (infected needles, syringes, surgical instruments, multidose vials, etc.) or the level of contamination in certain areas of the hospital.
     - Environmental cultures, including screening of healthcare personnel, should not be done unless epidemiologic evidence clearly indicates an environmental source of the pathogen. However, if certain species of microorganisms (e.g., *S. aureus*, HBV, *S. pyogenes*) are involved, the possibility of a carrier should be taken into account [19].

5. *The suspected epidemiologic link should be confirmed by typing of the microbial isolate.*
   - Traditional typing systems based on phenotype, such as serotype, biotype, phage type, or antibiogram, have been used for many years.
   - Currently, a wide variety of genotype-based typing methods are available with very high discriminatory ability, which have revolutionized our ability to distinguish all epidemiologically unrelated isolates [20, 21]. Some of these methods are as follows:
     - Pulsed-field gel electrophoresis (PFGE).
     - Amplified fragment length polymorphism (AFLP).
     - Random amplification of polymorphic DNA (RAPD).
     - Repetitive-element PCR (rep-PCR).
     - Variable-number tandem repeat (VNTR) typing.

- Multilocus VNTR analysis (MLVA).
- Single-locus sequence typing (SLST).
- Multilocus sequence typing (MLST).
- Whole genome sequencing (WGS).
- The choice of an appropriate molecular typing method (or methods) depends significantly on the problem to solve and the epidemiological context in which the method is going to be used.
- The microbiology laboratory should decide which of the typing tests it can do reliably on site and which should be sent to appropriate reference laboratories.
- Ideally the method used must be rapid, inexpensive, highly reproducible, and easy to perform and interpret. Additionally, a typing method used for surveillance should rely on an internationally standardized nomenclature, should be portable, and should be applicable for a broad range of bacterial species [20].
- Unfortunately, there is currently no single ideal typing method available, and each approach has various advantages and disadvantages [20, 21].

6. A *clonal outbreak* suggests a point source or nosocomial transmission, in which case a *case-control study should be performed*, comparing infected patients of the same age, gender, and service with exposure to potential risk factors.

7. Continue surveillance to document the efficacy of control measures.

8. Summarize the investigation in a written report to communicate findings.

9. The ICC should review infection control policies related to the outbreak depending on the agent and mode of transmission as revise if necessary.

References

1. World Health Organization. World alliance for patient safety: global patient safety challenge2005–2006. 2005. Availablefrom: http://www.who.int/patient-safety/events/05/HH_en.pdf

2. Pittet D, Allegranzi B, Storr J, Donaldson L. 'Clean Care is Safer Care': the global patient safety challenge 2005–2006. Int J Infect Dis. 2006;10(6):419–24. Epub 2006/08/18.

3. Mitchell DH, Swift G, Gilbert GL. Surgical wound infection surveillance: the importance of infections that develop after hospital discharge. Aust N Z J Surg. 1999;69(2):117–20. Epub 1999/02/25.

4. Prospero E, Cavicchi A, Bacelli S, Barbadoro P, Tantucci L, D'Errico MM. Surveillance for surgical site infection after hospital discharge: a surgical procedure-specific perspective. Infect Control Hosp Epidemiol. 2006;27(12):1313–17. Epub 2006/12/08.

5. Holtz TH, Wenzel RP. Postdischarge surveillance for nosocomial wound infection: a brief review and commentary. Am J Infect Control. 1992;20(4):206–13. Epub 1992/08/01.

6. World Health Organization. The global patient safety challenge 2005–2006 "Clean Care is Safer Care". 2005. Available from: http://www.who.int/patient-safety/events/05/GPSC_Launch_ENGLISH_FINAL.pdf

7. Harbarth S, Sax H, Gastmeier P. The preventable proportion of nosocomial infections: an overview of published reports. J Hosp Infect. 2003;54(4):258–66. quiz 321. Epub 2003/08/16.

8. Emori TG, Gaynes RP. An overview of nosocomial infections, including the role of the microbiology laboratory. Clin Microbiol Rev. 1993;6(4):428–42. Epub 1993/10/01.

9. Ducel G. JF, Nicolle L. Prevention of hospital-acquired infections. A practical guide. Available from: http://www.who.int/…urces/publications/whocdscs-reph200212.pdf

10. Cook E, Marchaim D, Kaye KS. Building a successful infection prevention program: key components, processes, and economics. Infect Dis Clin North Am. 2011;25(1):1–19. Epub 2011/02/15.

11. Murphy DM. From expert data collectors to interventionists: changing the focus for infection control professionals. Am J Infect Control. 2002;30(2):120–32. Epub 2002/04/11.

12. Pittet D. Clean hands reduce the burden of disease. Lancet. 2005;366(9481):185–7. Epub 2005/07/19.

13. Sarma JB, Ahmed GU. Infection control with limited resources: why and how to make it possible? Indian J Med Microbiol. 2010;28(1):11–6. Epub 2010/01/12.

14. Haley RW, Culver DH, White JW, Morgan WM, Emori TG, Munn VP, et al. The efficacy of infection surveillance and control programs in preventing nosocomial infections in US hospitals. Am J Epidemiol. 1985;121(2):182–205. Epub 1985/02/01.

15. Damani N. Simple measures save lives: an approach to infection control in countries with limited resources. J Hosp Infect. 2007;65 Suppl 2:151–4. Epub 2007/08/19.

16. McGrath EJ, Asmar BI. Nosocomial infections and multidrug-resistant bacterial organisms in the pediatric intensive care unit. Indian J Pediatr. 2011;78(2):176–84. Epub 2010/10/12.

17. Lee SC, Wu MS, Shih HJ, Huang SH, Chiou MJ, See LC, et al. Identification of vancomycin-resistant enterococci clones and inter-hospital spread during an outbreak in Taiwan. BMC Infect Dis. 2013;13:163. Epub 2013/04/06.

18. Guidelines for prevention of nosocomial pneumonia. Centers for Disease Control and Prevention. MMWR recommendations and reports: morbidity and mortality weekly report Recommendations and reports/Centers for Disease Control. 1997;46(RR-1):1–79. Epub 1997/01/03.

19. Danzmann L, Gastmeier P, Schwab F, Vonberg RP. Health care workers causing large nosocomial outbreaks: a systematic review. BMC Infect Dis. 2013;13:98. Epub 2013/02/26.

20. Sabat AJ, Budimir A, Nashev D, Sa-Leao R, van Dijl J, Laurent F, et al. Overview of molecular typing methods for outbreak detection and epidemiological surveillance. Euro Surveill. 2013;18(4):20380.

21. van Belkum A, Tassios PT, Dijkshoorn L, Haeggman S, Cookson B, Fry NK, et al. Guidelines for the validation and application of typing methods for use in bacterial epidemiology. Clin Microbiol Infect. 2007;13 Suppl 3:1–46. Epub 2007/11/06.

The Role of Microbiology Laboratory in Infection Prevention

5

Erin Fortier and Nancy Khardori

Identification of the etiologic agents and assessment of antimicrobial susceptibility patterns of significant bacterial isolates are the two primary responsibilities of microbiology laboratory. The increase of antibiotic resistance has become a serious global issue. Infections caused by drug-resistant bacteria are associated with increased morbidity, mortality, and of course higher healthcare-related costs. Over the past few decades, the inappropriate use of antibiotics has created "superbugs" which once considered a rare find in the Microbiology Laboratory are now seen daily. In any bacterial population, there are a proportion of bacteria with natural resistance to a given antibiotic. If that antibiotic is used for too long or too frequently, the resistant bacteria will selectively reproduce, and a phenotypic resistance to the antibiotic will emerge. It is not the use of the antibiotic but, rather, the misuse that results in resistance [1]. Physicians need to educate their patient on when antibiotics are to be used or not and if prescribed the appropriate use of the antibiotic and how noncompliance will create resistance further down the road. Unfortunately, antibiotic prescribing has become the path of "least resistance" and least time commitment for the medical profession at large.

In assisting physicians with what antibiotics are useful against specific organisms, the antibiogram report generated by the Microbiology Laboratory is an essential tool in addition to monitoring trends in drug resistance in their particular healthcare facility. The cumulative antibiogram report is a summary of susceptibility rates for particular organisms. The M39-A2 consensus document from the Clinical and Laboratory Standards Institute (CLSI) entitled "Analysis and Presentation of Cumulative Antimicrobial Susceptibility Test Data" provides guidance to clinical laboratories in the preparation of a cumulative antibiogram. The most frequent use of a cumulative antibiogram report is in guiding initial empirical/presumptive antimicrobial therapy decisions for the management of infections prior to availability of microbiological test results, and this is the focus of CLSI M39-A2 [2]. Early eradication of the infecting organism and prevention of further antibiotic resistance have a significant impact on transmission and therefore infection prevention.

Due to the worldwide increase of antimicrobial resistance, there is a real need to monitor any trends that could be emerging at the local level. In the year 2000, a survey coordinated by the Clinical and Laboratory Standards Institute highlighted the diversity of calculation algorithms used in the clinical laboratories in the United States (data not published). Two observations from the survey were as follows: (1) there may be poor comparability of antimicrobial susceptibility

E. Fortier, MLS (ASCP)
Bon Secours De Paul Medical Center, Norfolk, VA, USA

N. Khardori, M.D., Ph.D. (✉)
Division of Infectious Diseases, Department of Internal Medicine, Eastern Virginia Medical School, Norfolk, VA, USA

Department of Microbiology and Molecular Cell Biology, Eastern Virginia Medical School, Norfolk, VA, USA
e-mail: nkhardori@gmail.com

Table 5.1 Cumulative antibiogram provided by the Microbiology Department for the Bon Secours System which located in Virginia

Organism	# isolates	Amikacin	Ampicillin	Ampicillin/sulbactam	Aztreonam	Cefazolin	Cefepime	Ceftazidime	Ceftriaxone	Cefotetan	Ciprofloxacin	Clindamycin
Gram-negative												
Escherichia coli	715	100	43–50	54–63	91–94	84–88	93–96	90–93	91–93	99		
Klebsiella pneumoniae	306	81–100	0	68–90	73–100	72–94	73–100	73–98	73–100	75–100		
Enterobacter cloacae	95	98–100			78–97	0	90–100	73–79	72–73	0		
Proteus mirabilis	243	100	52–83	76–89	95–100	76–90	99–100	95–99	97–100	100		
Acinetobacter baumannii	53	50–75		25–95	0		17–73	8–67	0–11			
Pseudomonas aeruginosa	341	98–100			60–64		86–92	83–89	1–2			
Gram-positive												
Streptococcus pneumoniae (fluid)	3								66[a]			
Streptococcus pneumoniae (non-fluid)	27								86–100[a]			
Enterococcus faecalis	426		96–99								58–72	
Enterococcus faecium	70		17–35									
Staphylococcus aureus	814			42–50		41–50						64–76
Staphylococcus epidermidis	316			22–34		22–34						45–71

Note: antibiotics may have a range of susceptibility due to the data obtained from a system that
[a]based on new breakpoints for ceftriaxone for non-meningitis isolates of *S. pneumoniae*
[b]Rifampin/gentamicin should not be used alone for therapy

consists of three facilities, Maryview Medical Center, DePaul Medical Center, and Mary Immaculate Hospital

Erythromycin	Gentamicin	Levofloxacin	Meropenem	Oxacillin	Nitrofurantoin	Synercid	Penicillin G	Linezolid	Tetracycline	Tigecycline	Trimethoprim/sulfamethox.	Vancomycin	Gentamicin synergy[b]	Streptomycin synergy
	88–91	53–68	100		93–95						72–81			
	90–100	71–98	75–100		34–43						81–96			
	96–100	80–100	90–100								86–100			
	90–97	38–70	100	0							57–82			
	17–80	15–73	0–30								17–73			
	81–96	55–69	83–95								0			
		100					0					100		
14–83		100					43–80		43–100		71–100	100		
		64–73			96–100		96–99		20–22			98–99	68–79	70–80
		7–14				100	17–35	92–100	8–21			39–45	89–97	69–96
28–72	98[b]	46–57		41–50			0		95–98	100	95–98	100		
29–38	76[b]	27–42		22–34			0		81–96	100	36–49	100		

statistics between institutions because of the diversity of calculations methods, and (2) many laboratories use a simplistic calculations approach, with a strong tendency to overestimate drug-resistance rates [3]. The CLSI M39-A2 document has specific recommendations on how laboratories are to collect and report their findings.

First that the Microbiology Laboratory collect a year's worth of susceptibility data based on Minimum Inhibitory Concentration or MIC for the report, larger facilities can generate a report more frequently and whenever there is a change in the susceptibility of certain organisms during the year. It is also recommended that >30 isolates of species encountered be reported; for smaller facilities, it may be necessary to combine more than a year's worth of data, but that information must be noted on the report. Isolates that are tested for surveillance must not be counted in the antibiogram as they are generally only for screening purposes and not in the group of organisms recovered that are tested against antibiotics for treatment. Repeat isolates should be discounted. Recommendations also include that only antibiotics routinely tested and reported be included in the report. The "off-line" agents that are specifically asked to be tested for individual patients should not be included. The report will show the percentage of isolates that are susceptible to the particular antibiotic that is routinely tested against that organism in that particular facility. The antibiogram can differ in what antibiotics are routinely tested within an area because facilities may have chosen different panels to run based on recommendations from pharmacy and infectious disease practitioners. These panels of antibiotics are set by various manufacturers and cannot vary due to each physician's preference. CLSI recommends that the antibiogram be published either on the facility's website for easy access by all clinicians or in pocket guides. The report should also be distributed to the pharmacy as well as the infection prevention department.

The data in the report is specific for that particular facility and can assist the clinician in choosing empirical/presumptive therapy while waiting for laboratory results on an individual patient's organism. Since the first 48–72 h is the most crucial time period to morbidity and mortality from a serious infectious process, the selection of initial presumptive antimicrobial therapy is the single most step in management. In this sense, if the patient improves with the initial selection, the subsequent culture and susceptibility results become useful for the second step of de-escalating and streamlining antimicrobial therapy. Both of these interventions have significant positive impact on antimicrobial resistance, cost, and infection prevention. Continuation of initial broad-spectrum antibiotic regimens even a targeted "Magic bullet" can be substituted is a common practice. This approach broadens the extent of collateral damage to the resident flora and creates an environment for development of resistance.

This report when reviewed annually can easily show the trends that the facility has towards increased resistance for a particular organism against a certain antibiotic. The Microbiology Laboratory can choose to prepare the report quarterly for review of trends but present the report annually. The Microbiology Laboratory should notify the infection prevention and the pharmacy departments during the monthly or quarterly meetings followed by sending alerts to the clinicians.

Currently there is no standardization among facilities when it comes to the process of generating the report. It is a requirement for the report to be generated by those laboratories that are accredited by the College of American Pathologists (CAP) and to distribute the report within the facility. Table 5.1 shows a typical antibiogram generated by three hospital microbiology laboratories at a hospital system on Hampton Roads, Virginia. The report divides the bacteria into gram-positive and gram-negative groups. The organisms shown have at least 30 isolates for the year, and the listed antibiotics are routinely tested at the system. Other antibiotics are available for testing per specific requests but are not a part of the calculations.

The numbers listed represent a particular organism's percentage of susceptible isolates to that particular antibiotic. For example, there were 715 isolates of *E. coli* recovered in the year, and 72–81 % of those isolates were susceptible to trimethoprim-sulfamethoxazole, whereas only 43–50 % were susceptible to ampicillin. The physicians using this chart can then choose trimethoprim- sulfamethoxazole over ampicillin to treat infections known to be commonly caused by *E. coli* prior to results becoming available on a given patient. The cumulative report gives the prescribers the option of focusing on the agents with highest susceptibility rates and choosing among them the best suited to a particular patient based on the route needed, pharmacokinetics, pharmacodynamics, comorbidities, and other host-related factors. The Microbiology Laboratory can provide further assistance by detection of various types of beta lactamases, the presence of which compounds the problems associated with selection of antimicrobial therapy [4]. More specialized and complex testing such as Minimum Bactericidal Concentration (MBC), Time-Kill Kinetic assay, Serum Inhibitory and Bactericidal concentration, and synergy testing are available in larger laboratories and reference laboratories for difficult-to-treat infections [5]. It is the responsibility of the laboratory to make prescribers aware of these options.

Recent Developments

Molecular diagnostic testing developed recently provides a sensitive, specific, and timely/real-time tool for active surveillance-driven infection prevention interventions. The turnaround time with these tests is such that they potentially support point-of-care decision making. Table 5.2 lists the currently FDA-approved molecular diagnostics for nosocomial pathogens. The initial investment in the equipment may be the biggest hurdle for smaller laboratories. However, laboratory-based decisions on the cost of testing do not take into account the downstream cost effect from inappropriate isolation measures, barrier precautions, and unreimbursed nosocomial infections. A recent study strongly suggested that the increased cost of real-time PCR testing for *C. difficile* would be more than offset by its impact on the downstream costs associated with the use of current less sensitive tests resulting in unnecessary repeat testing, isolation and barrier precautions, unnecessary antibiotic use, and inadequate infection prevention [6]. In the United States, Centers for Disease Control and Prevention and Society for Healthcare

Table 5.2 Molecular diagnostics useful for infection prevention currently approved by FDA

Assay type	Target pathogen	Turnaround time
1 Real-time PCR	*C. difficile, S. aureus,* MRSA, VRE	1.5 h[a]
2 Real-time PCR	*C. difficile, S. aureus,* MRSA, VRE	1 h[a]
3 Isothermic DNA Amplification	*C. difficile*	1 h
4 Real-time PCR	*C. difficile*	3–4 h
5 Real-time PCR	MRSA	2 h
6 Real-time PCR	MRSA	2 h

[a]High-throughput platform

Epidemiology suggest implementing targeting active surveillance programs when traditional infection control activities have been unsuccessful in controlling multidrug-resistant pathogens. Such interventions generally target high-risk populations or areas and require highly sensitive screening tests with short turnaround times [7]. The rapid molecular screening tests are most suited especially the ones that offer high throughput platforms to facilitate large volume testing and kits that target a number of pathogens.

References

1. Davies PDO. Does increased use of antibiotics result in increased antibiotic resistance. Clin Infect Dis. 2004;39:18–9.
2. Clinical and Laboratory Standards Institute (CLSI). Analysis and presentation of cumulative antimicrobial susceptibility test data, Approved guideline M39-A2. 2nd ed. Wayne: CLSI; 2006.
3. Hindler JF, Steriling J. Analysis and presentation of cumulative antibiograms: a new consensus guideline from the Clinical and Laboratory Standards Institute. Clin Infect Dis. 2007;44:867–73.
4. Jenkins SG, Schultz AN. Current concepts in laboratory testing to guide antimicrobial therapy. Mayo Clinic Proc. 2012;87(3):290–308.
5. Jenkins SG, Jerris RC. Critical assessment of issues applicable to development of antimicrobial susceptibility testing break points. J Clin Microbiol. 2011;49(9 suppl):S5–14.
6. Curris B. PCR testing to improve patient outcomes and reduce C. difficile associated cost. Mang Infect Control. 2009:94–97.
7. Diekema D, Endona M. Look before you leap: active surveillance for multidrug resistant organisms. Clin Infect Dis. 2007;44(8):1101–7.

Role of Antimicrobial Stewardship in Infection Prevention

6

Thomas J. Lynch, Erin Fortier, Divya Trehan, and Nancy Khardori

Introduction

Since the 1980s, there has been a widespread and inappropriate use of antimicrobials in our hospitals. This started in part due to the continual development and marketing of an ever-expanding array of drugs to replace agents that would quickly lose their effectiveness secondary to development of resistance. As antimicrobials began to consume a significant percentage of the hospital pharmacy budget, some hospitals developed antimicrobial management or control programs in an attempt to primarily reduce direct drug costs. These early programs have now evolved into antimicrobial stewardship programs (ASPs) which attempt to also improve the quality and appropriateness of antimicrobial use. The concept of stewardship implies an obligation for responsible management of resources. Today high costs of antimicrobials still persist and are estimated to account for 30 %

of a hospital budget [1]. However, costs are now only part of a much larger issue. There has been a dramatic increase in antimicrobial resistance in response to constant antimicrobial exposure in institutions. New drugs effective against resistant strains are in short supply, can have significant toxicity, and can be extremely expensive. Resistance has, in turn, led to increases in length of stay with high indirect healthcare costs. The problem has become so pervasive that the Infectious Disease Society of America (IDSA) has recently recommended that ASPs be required in all acute care hospitals in the United States [2]. ASPs are already obligatory in the United Kingdom and the European Union. As a corollary to minimizing expansion of antimicrobial resistance, ASPs reduce the transmission of resistant bacteria in the hospital setting and the requirement for expensive "isolation measures" and therefore have a significant role in infection prevention.

T.J. Lynch, PharmD (✉)
Eastern Virginia Medical School, Norfolk, VA, USA
e-mail: nlyncht@evms.edu

E. Fortier, MLS(ASCP) • D. Trehan, PharmD
Bon Secours De Paul Medical Center, Norfolk
VA, USA

N. Khardori, M.D., Ph.D.
Division of Infectious Diseases, Department
of Internal Medicine, Eastern Virginia Medical School,
Norfolk, VA, USA

Department of Microbiology and Molecular Cell
Biology, Eastern Virginia Medical School,
Norfolk, VA, USA
e-mail: nkhardori@gmail.com

ASP Goals

The primary goal of ASPs is to improve clinical outcomes while minimizing adverse events secondary to antimicrobial use, such as the development of resistance and/or toxicity. This is accomplished by implementing and managing strategies that optimize the appropriate selection, dosing, route, and duration of antimicrobial therapy at an institution. It has been estimated that up to 50 % of antimicrobial use was inappropriate in institutions before establishment of ASPs [3].

C. Wattal and N. Khardori (eds.), *Hospital Infection Prevention: Principles & Practices*,
DOI 10.1007/978-81-322-1608-7_6, © Springer India 2014

The ASP Interdisciplinary Team

Ideally, an interdisciplinary team should be established to develop and manage an ASP. At a minimum, the team should include an infectious disease physician specialist and a clinical pharmacist with specialized training or certification in infectious diseases. Other critical team members could include representatives of the microbiology laboratory, infection control service, information technology, and hospital administration. Most often the pharmacist performs the day-to-day activities of an ASP such as guideline development, education, and pre- and post-antimicrobial order review [4].

Potential ASP Strategies

Recently, the Infectious Disease Society of America and the Society for Healthcare Epidemiology of America jointly published evidence-based guidelines for developing and managing ASPs in healthcare institutions [5]. Prior to implementing specific APS strategies, it is essential to develop institution-specific antimicrobial use guidelines and then implement an educational program to disseminate these guidelines. Then, as discussed by Dellit et al. [5], there are two core strategies that provide the foundation for most successful antimicrobial stewardship programs. The first is prospective auditing of antimicrobial use with intervention and direct feedback to the prescriber by a member of the ASP interdisciplinary team (usually an ID physician or a clinical pharmacist). The authors gave this approach the highest rating for effectiveness (A-1) based on the results of multiple controlled trials. This strategy is employed after an antimicrobial is dispensed and can target a specific population or drug. The intervention can be either verbal or in writing and its effectiveness can be enhanced by use of computer surveillance.

The second core strategy is the use of formulary restriction and preauthorization requirements. This method has been effective in quickly getting antimicrobial expenditures under control and can result in significant savings in direct drug costs. However, there is less evidence that this method can result in a significant change in antimicrobial resistance patterns. Also, prospectively restricting the use of one antimicrobial can lead to the increased and inappropriate use of alternative antimicrobials, unless overall antimicrobial use trends are also monitored. Restriction can refer to the authorized use of only certain antimicrobials in an institution. Or, more commonly, it refers to the use of an antimicrobial for an established set of criteria. These criteria can be taken from national guidelines or developed locally by the ASP interdisciplinary team and/or the Pharmacy and Therapeutics Committee. The effectiveness of a preauthorization program can depend on who is responsible for screening requests and making recommendations. Greater compliance with recommendations is likely if the policies are approved by a hospital's medical executive committee. In a randomized comparison of the two core strategies at a large teaching hospital, Camins et al. [6] found that prospective audit and feedback was associated with a shorter median duration of inappropriate antimicrobial use (2 vs. 5 days), a lower median antimicrobial defined daily dose (2 vs. 4 DDD), and a slightly shorter median duration of length of stay (7 vs. 8 days).

Besides the two core strategies reviewed by Dellit et al. [5], there are several supplemental strategies that are discussed and graded based on published evidence of efficacy. Those that had good evidence to support a recommendation (Grade A) included education programs, as an element of an overall core strategy, to increase the effectiveness of an ASP; the development of guidelines and clinical pathways incorporating local microbiology results and resistance patterns to improve antimicrobial utilization; streamlining empirical/presumptive therapy on the basis of culture results to decrease both antimicrobial pressure and direct drug costs; optimization of dosing based on individual patient characteristics, site of infection, and causative organism; and systematic parenteral to oral dose conversion to decrease length of stay and healthcare costs.

Those strategies that had moderate evidence to support recommendation included education programs *not* linked to an ASP core strategy and use of an antimicrobial order form, in conjunction with restrictive criteria, to decrease inappropriate use of antimicrobials at the point of prescribing. Strategies that had poor evidence to support recommendation included automatic substitution of one antimicrobial for another (cycling) to theoretically cause a reduction in selection pressure and antimicrobial resistance to the restricted agent and use of antimicrobial combinations specifically to prevent emergence of resistance.

If personnel and financial resources are limited, such as at smaller hospitals, Goff et al. [7] suggest some interventions where targets can be more easily obtained ("low-hanging fruit"). These include parenteral to oral conversion, batching of expensive intravenous antimicrobials when preparing doses for dispensing, therapeutic substitutions, and formulary restriction. Several antibiotic classes have great oral bioavailability which allows for intravenous to oral switch when appropriate. This cuts down on drug cost while providing therapy of equal efficacy and reduces the rate of intravenous line – related complications including septicemia. Computerized alerts can assist in notifying appropriate persons/teams when criteria are met for a switch. In the United States, 120 Veterans Affairs hospitals reported a cost savings of four million dollars between 2006 and 2010 by converting intravenous formulations of fluoroquinolones to oral whenever feasible [7]. Developing ways for the pharmacy to prepare drugs in ways that minimize waste especially for "high dollar" antimicrobials is another tool to reduce cost. At the Ohio State University Wexner Medical Center, the pharmacy department prepare all the orders for daptomycin and caspofungin at a specified time each day in a sterile hood. It altered the times the first and second doses were given; however, the facility had an annual cost avoidance of $ 60,000 for caspofungin and $ 250,000 for daptomycin [7].

Documentation of Processes and Outcomes of ASPs

Once ASP strategies have been put into place, it is necessary to establish and measure both processes and outcomes according to Khadem et al. [8]. Process measures answer whether the intervention strategy resulted in the desired change in antimicrobial utilization. Outcome measures reflect expected changes in clinical outcome such as infection-related mortality, length of hospital stay, rates of readmission, and antimicrobial resistance rates. Both process and outcome measures need to be defined for any ASP strategy to confirm that goals of the intervention were attained and clinical objectives met. This is also necessary if the ASP team wishes to receive continued financial support from hospital administration.

Steps for Planning and Implementation of an ASP

For institutions contemplating the development or enhancement of an ASP, Tamma and Cosgrove [9] have provided a step-by-step process that should be employed. This is particularly important when approaching hospital administration for support of an ASP:

Step 1: Frame the problem that needs to be targeted.

Step 2: Consider potential solutions to the problem.

Step 3: Decide what needs to occur to achieve the solutions.

Step 4: Meet key administrative leaders to determine if the issue is of institutional concern and if they will give their support.

Step 5: Estimate the annual costs, which may include added personnel and extra computer support.

Step 6: Determine the costs associated with the infection of interest.

Step 7: Calculate the financial effect of the intervention (estimated cost savings minus costs needed in advance).

Step 8: Include any additional benefits, such as improved clinical outcomes, as evidenced by the literature.

Step 9: Prospectively collect process and outcome data.

Conclusion

Effective antimicrobial stewardship programs require an interdisciplinary team approach that incorporates many strategic elements at the same time. At the core of effective programs should be a proactive strategy incorporating prospective audits of selected antimicrobial prescribing with direct intervention and feedback to the provider as well as preauthorization requirements and formulary restriction [5]. Studies of the clinical and economic impact of ASPs consistently demonstrate a decrease in inappropriate antimicrobial use and annual savings of $200,000–$900,000 in both large academic hospitals and small community hospitals [5]. Stewardship of antimicrobial use in our institutions and community is essential now more than ever to preserve the effectiveness of a dwindling array of antimicrobial agents as the pharmaceutical industry continues to reduce its investment in the research, development, and production of new agents.

As the burden of multidrug-resistant bacteria lightens, so will the requirement for "isolation measures" and the overall rate of transmission of such organisms in the hospital setting.

References

1. John JF, Fishman NO. Programmatic role of the infectious disease physician in controlling antimicrobial costs in the hospital. Clin Infect Dis. 1997;24:471–85.
2. Infectious Disease Society of America. Infection prevention and control of health care-associated infection. http://www.idsociety.org/Infection_Control_Policy/. Accessed 16 April 2013.
3. Marr JJ, Moffet HI, Kunin CM. Guidelines for improving the use of antimicrobial agents in hospitals: a statement of the Infectious Disease Society of America. J Infect Dis. 1988;157:869–76.
4. Drew RH, White R, MacDougall C, et al. Insights from the Society of Infectious Disease Pharmacists on antimicrobial stewardship guidelines from the Infectious Disease Society of America and the Society for Healthcare Epidemiology of America. Pharmacotherapy. 2009;29:593–607.
5. Dellit TH, Owens RC, McGowan Jr JE, et al. Infectious Diseases Society of America and the Society for Healthcare Epidemiology of America guidelines for developing an institutional program to enhance antimicrobial stewardship. Clin Infect Dis. 2007;44:159–77.
6. Camins BC, King MD, Wells JB, et al. Impact of an antimicrobial utilization program on antimicrobial use at a large teaching hospital: a randomized controlled trial. Infect Control Hosp Epidemiol. 2009;30:931–8.
7. Goff DA, Bauer KA, Reed EE, et al. Is the "Low-Hanging Fruit" worth picking for antimicrobial stewardship programs? Clin Infect Dis. 2012;55:587–92.
8. Khadem TM, Ashley ED, Wrobel MJ, Brown J. Antimicrobial stewardship: a matter of process or outcome? Pharmacotherapy. 2012;32:688–706.
9. Tamma PD, Cosgrove SE. Antimicrobial stewardship. Infect Dis Clin N Am. 2011;25:245–60.

A Four-Step Approach to Antibiotic Stewardship in India: Formulation of Antibiotic Policy

Chand Wattal and J.K. Oberoi

The four main steps [1, 2] for formulation of an antibiotic policy include the following:

1. Step one: Compile local hospital data based on site of infection (Jan–Dec of X year). Validity of these data: Dec X + 1 year
   - Demographic variations (ICUs/wards/surgical site infections, etc.)
   - *% Distribution of bugs*
   - *% Susceptibility to antibiotics*
2. Step two: Identify the five most common pathogens isolated.
3. Step three: Identify the five most sensitive antibiotics.
4. Step four: Define patient type (*risk stratification for each patient's type* (Table 7.1)).
5. Based on the above data, a presumptive antibiotic policy can be formulated, an example of which is shown in Fig. 7.1.

Type 4 patient can also be added in special circumstances with suspicion of fungal (Candida) infection.

Type 4: Description

Type 3 patient with fever despite antibiotic therapy (> 5 days) with no obvious source/after appropriate source control ± severe sepsis/septic shock PLUS

Has ≥ 1 of the following risk factors (but not limited to) for invasive fungal infections:
- TPN
- Hemodialysis
- Immunodeficiency of variable origin
- Major abdominal surgery
- Multifocal Candida colonization
- Diabetes

Suggested protocol for Type 4 patient:
- If hemodynamically stable and no prior exposure to Azoles – fluconazole
- If hemodynamically stable but with prior exposure to Azoles – echinocandins/Lip Amp B/Conv. Amp B[1]
- If hemodynamically unstable – echinocandins/Lip Amp B

C. Wattal, M.D. (✉) • J.K. Oberoi, M.D.
Department of Clinical Microbiology, Sir Ganga Ram Hospital, New Delhi, India
e-mail: chandwattal@gmail.com

[1]Consider de-escalation to Azoles after seeing patient condition and culture/sensitivity report.

Table 7.1 Risk stratification for patient type

	Type 1	Type 2	Type 3
Health-care contact	No	Yes	Prolonged
Procedures	No	Minimum	Major invasive procedures
Antibiotic treatment history	No in last 90 days	Yes in last 90 days	Repeat multiple antibiotics
Patient characteristics	Young, no comorbid conditions	Elderly, few comorbid conditions	Immunocompromised +/−, many comorbid conditions
Possible pathogen	Susceptible to common narrow spectrum antibiotics	ESBLs//MRSA	ESBLs + Pseudomonas + MRSA

Blood Stream Infections (BSIs) Antibiotic Protocol: ICU (*valid upto June,2009*)

ICU MICROBIOLOGY DATA (*Total no. of isolates = 171*)

Most Common Pathogens	%	Antibiotics Susceptibility	%
Acinetobacter (n=48)	28%	Colistin / Imipenem (=Amikacin) / Cef/Sul / Piptazo	98%; 9%; 6%; 2%
Klebsiella (n=43)	25%	Imipenem (~Ertapenem) / Amikacin / Piptazo / Cef/Sul	97%; 43%; 33%; 21%
E.coli (n=24)	14%	Imipenem (~Ertapenem) / Amikacin / Piptazo (=Cef/Sul)	100%; 92%; 67%
Pseudomonas (n=20)	12%	Colistin / Pip/Taz / Imipenem / Cef/Sul (=Amikacin)	91%; 62%; 29%; 27%
Staph CNS(n=16)	9%	Vancomycin (~Teicoplanin)	100%

Patient Type 1 (CAI)	Patient Type 2 (HAI)	Patient Type 3 (NI)
No contact with health care system	Contact with health care system (e.g. recent hospital admission, nursing home, dialysis) without invasive procedure	Long hospitalization and or invasive procedures
No prior antibiotic treatment	Recent antibiotic therapy	Recent & multiple antibiotic therapies
Patient young with few co-morbid conditions	Patient old with multiple co-morbidities.	Cystic fibrosis, structural lung disease, advanced AIDS, neutropenia, other severe immunodeficiency.
Send Sample for Culture	*Send Sample for Culture*	*Send Sample for Culture*
PRESUMPTIVE THERAPY	**PRESUMPTIVE THERAPY**	**PRESUMPTIVE THERAPY**
Ampicillin/ Ampicillin-sulbactam/ Amoxi-Clavulanate Ceftriaxone Ciprofloxacin*	Ertapenem/Tigecycline** ± Vancomycin/ Teicoplanin	Colistin+Imipenem+Sulbactam ± Vancomycin or teicoplanin
After Culture Report	**After Culture Report**	**After Culture Report**
Continue Treatment	**Continue Treatment**	**Continue Treatment**
S.typhi: Continue the treatment	ESBL +ve Klebsiella / E.coli: Continue treatment with monotherapy	Susceptible PA/AB /MRSA. Continue treatment as monotherapy
Stop "De-Escalate "	**Stop "De-Escalate "**	**Stop "De-Escalate "**
Continue monotherapy	Non ESBL Enterobacteriaceae, De-Escalate & Treat it as patients type 1	ESBL Positive Enterobacteriaceae, De-Escalate and treat as Patients Type 2
Consider Escalation	**Consider Escalation**	**Consider Escalation**
ESBL +ve Enterobacteriaceae including Salmonella: Escalate and treat as patient type 2	PA/AB: Escalate and treat as Patient Type 3; in case of MRSA add Vancomycin or Teicoplanin	MDR-PA or AB. Continue 3 Drug Colistin + Imipenem + Sulbactam

*Avoid Ciprofloxacin since it has potent antipesudomonal activity

Fig. 7.1 An antibiotic policy for bloodstream infections (BSI) based on local hospital data

In case of proven or probable cases of aspergillosis, voriconazole/L Amp B is preferred.

Note: Febrile neutropenia needs to be viewed separately.

References

1. Microbiology newsletter. Sir Ganga Ram Hospital. Available at. http://www.sgrh.com/publications.php. Accessed 31 May 2013.
2. National policy for Containment of Antimicrobial resistance India. Available at. http://www.ncdc.gov.in/ab_policy.pdf. Accessed 31 May 2013.

Part VI

Role of Hospital Housekeeping and Materials Management Including Disinfection and Waste Management

Role of Hospital Housekeeping and Materials Management Including Disinfection and Waste Management

8

Purva Mathur

Cleaning of Hospital Surfaces

Introduction

Pathogens are shed on hospital surfaces and aerosolized continuously in all patient care areas. Hospital surfaces thus constitute a major reservoir of potentially pathogenic and resistant organisms. Proper and regular cleaning of housekeeping (non-critical) surfaces reduces this reservoir and also provides an aesthetically pleasing environment. Cleaning of health-care facilities is performed for medical and sociocultural reasons. Maintaining an environment with a low microbial burden is required to avoid complications during the care and recovery of patients. Moreover, a healthy, safe, and aesthetically pleasing environment in a health-care facility with clean surfaces is comforting to patients, their families, and visitors by giving an impression of good quality care without additional health hazards. Clean surroundings are also soothing for the health-care workers. The cleaning procedures should be such that they reduce aerosolization and the bio-burden of pathogens from hospital surfaces. The cleaning products should be safe, environment-friendly, and effective to reduce the pathogenic contamination of hospital surfaces.

Thus, health-care settings require intensive and frequent cleaning with a wide range of products.

The environment in a hospital usually refers to the patient's surroundings. Thus, cleaning the environment generally refers to cleaning and disinfecting objects like housekeeping surfaces (e.g., floors, tabletops, door handles, bed rails) and medical equipment. It is especially essential to focus on cleaning and disinfecting frequently touched items, such as bedrails, tray tables, side tables, doorknobs and handles, IV poles, call buttons, monitor screens, controls and cables, pump controls, bedside tables, telephones, carts, toilets, bedpans, sinks, light switches, TV remotes, and faucet handles.

The effectiveness of cleaning and disinfection to prevent transmission of pathogens to patients from environment depends on many factors like the nature of the object/surface/equipment; the type, number, and location of microorganisms; the capacity of the microbes to resist the disinfectants; the presence of organic and inorganic matter; the type of disinfectants; the concentration and potency of disinfectant; other physical and chemical properties (i.e., temperature, pH); the duration of exposure; and the contact time. Cleaning and disinfection of environment and housekeeping areas is just one of several steps needed to prevent the spread of germs.

The housekeeping surfaces and other environmental surfaces should be cleaned and disinfected regularly, when spills occur, and when these surfaces are visibly dirty. Some areas like

P. Mathur, M.D. (✉)
Department of Laboratory Medicine, JPNA Trauma Centre, AIIMS, New Delhi, India
e-mail: purvamathur@yahoo.co.in

ICUs, OTs, HDUs, and isolation rooms need more frequent cleaning.

Cleaning Procedures

The schedule and frequency of cleaning and disinfecting the environmental surfaces depends on many factors. Primary among this is the type of patient care area: high risk/postoperative/ICUs/HDUs/OTs/wards/laboratories/general areas, etc. The other factors are the type of surfaces, the amount of people's movement, and soiling [1, 2]. Since environmental surfaces are non-critical, the method of cleaning (to use a detergent or a germicide) remains a controversial subject, with no clear guideline [3–5]. The argument to use only detergent for routine cleaning is based on the fact that environmental surfaces contribute minimally to infections, and no difference in infection rates have been found if floors are cleaned with disinfectants as compared to detergents [1, 6–9]. Use of detergents is less costly and toxic and is also more environment-friendly. It is also argued that disinfectant-cleaned floors become rapidly contaminated with microorganisms after sometime. Therefore, the superiority of disinfection of floors is doubtful. However, detergents are less effective in reducing bacterial loads and become contaminated with bacteria [8]. Also, the use of disinfectants is recommended by CDC and OSHA for cleaning high-risk areas like isolation rooms, surfaces contaminated with blood or other infectious materials, and high-touch surfaces in the vicinity of patients shedding resistant pathogens like VRE and MRSA [6]. Moreover, the use of disinfectants also simplifies the training, implementation, and monitoring of a uniform cleaning protocol for the hospital and provides a margin for safety in cases of unconfirmed spills of infective material [6].

Each hospital should have a written protocol for cleaning and disinfection of surfaces and noncritical items. These should be followed and monitored by the hospital's Infection Control Committees. The hospital staff must be properly trained on the practices of cleaning and decontamination of hospital surfaces. Appropriate personal prophylactic equipments (PPE; gloves, masks, and boots) must be worn at all times, and a proper log of all cleaning procedures must be maintained [1, 2, 6, 10, 11]. The nurses in charge of the individual wards should keep a log of these procedures and take active part in training and monitoring of housekeeping staff. The hospital surfaces and frequently touched areas should be cleaned on a regular basis, when visibly soiled and when spills occur.

Cleaning may be done with detergent and hot water or an EPA-registered hospital disinfectant for housekeeping surfaces. Use of a low-/intermediate-level disinfectant is advocated in specific high-risk areas (ICUs, HDUs, transplant units, isolation rooms, areas housing immunocompromised patients, surgical suites, burns ward, OTs, emergency rooms, surfaces of dialysis machine, or when there is suspected spills of blood/body substances/MDR organisms). Disinfectants should not be used in offices. High-level disinfectants must not be used for environmental surfaces in any area of the hospital.

It is preferable to use a disinfectant registered by a competent government-approved agency. In the USA, disinfectants registered with the US Environmental Protection Agency (EPA) are used.

If the surface is visibly dirty, it should be cleaned before being disinfected. If the surface is not visibly dirty, a disinfecting wipe can be used on the surface or equipment. It is important to pay close attention to the directions for the disinfecting wipe and the contact time needed to be effective.

For general cleaning of housekeeping areas and surfaces, a recommended protocol is to prepare fresh detergent/disinfectant solutions every day, according to manufacturer's instructions, which should be replaced with fresh solution frequently. Disinfectants should be chosen by the hospital in consultation with the hospital's Infection Control Committee. The hospital's Infection Control Committee in turn should gather data regarding user acceptability from the various wards. Hospitals may select one EPA-registered disinfectant for all the wards, considering its activity, cost, safety, and material compatibility. At all times, the manufacturer's instructions should be followed for its use, dilution, period of use, storage, and disposal. Diluted disinfectants may become contaminated with resistant hospital pathogens, therefore, application of contaminated cleaning solution from spray bottles/equipment should be avoided, since they generate aerosols. The remaining solutions after day's use should be discarded, and the containers should be dried [1, 3–5, 7–9].

Dry mopping with brooms generate dust aerosols, therefore, it should be avoided in all patient care areas. Nonporous floors may be cleaned using vacuum cleaning, wet mopping, and dry dusting with electrostatic material and spray buffing. Ensure thorough physical wiping and scrubbing, which is as effective as the use of disinfectants in reducing the bio-burden. Wet dust horizontal surfaces daily with a clean cloth moistened with an EPA-registered hospital disinfectant (or detergent). The surfaces should be left dry after cleaning. Disinfectant fogging is not recommended for routine patient care areas [1, 3].

It is also important to reduce the contamination of cleaning agents and cleaning tools. Therefore, it is recommended to use a two-bucket system while doing wet mopping. When a single bucket is used, the solutions should be changed more frequently. The used cleaning solutions should be carefully discarded in the sluice. At the end of each cycle of cleaning, the buckets should be cleaned with detergent and warm water and store inverted to assist drying. Worn and damaged cleaning equipment should be replaced. It is preferable to use disposable mop heads, although they are costly and may not be suitable in resource limited situations. In such cases, mop heads should be changed after cleaning spills and at the beginning of the day. The mop heads and cleaning cloths should be decontaminated regularly to prevent contamination. This may be done by laundering (heat disinfection) with detergent and drying at 80 °C for 2 h daily or immersing the cloth in hypochlorite solution (4,000 ppm) for 2 min. Alternatively, dust-attracting mops (microfiber material) may be used, especially for critical care areas and high dependency units [1, 3, 4, 7–9].

The high-touch surfaces should be cleaned more frequently than minimally touched ones. The walls, blinds, and window curtains should be cleaned when they are visibly contaminated or soiled. Curtains in the vicinity of a disperser of epidemic MRSA strain may be changed if the area is to be re-occupied by a susceptible person within 24 h.

Recommended Cleaning Agents for Non-critical Items

The following agents are recommended by EPA for hard surface disinfection [12]:

Bleach (sodium hypochlorite; 5.25 %)

Phenols

Quaternary ammonium compounds

Accelerated hydrogen peroxide (hydrogen peroxide/anionic surfactants)

Botanicals (Benefect, e.g., Thymol)

Silver dihydrogen citrate (e.g., PureGreen24)

Most of these disinfectants require precleaning and belong to EPA toxicity categories I–IV. All these are low- or intermediate-level disinfectants. All except diluted bleach are stable on storage. Diluted bleach is stable only for 24 h. Most of them are effective against a broad spectrum of microbes, including influenza H1N1, and MRSA. Their dwell time is usually less than 10 min. However, many of these chemicals have adverse health effects. Therefore, manufacturer's recommendations must be strictly followed, and personal protective equipment must be worn to minimize exposure. The products must also be disposed according to manufacturer's instructions since they have environmental toxicity. An advantage of these products is that they are readily available and relatively inexpensive [12].

Cleaning of Spills

The following steps should be followed when cleaning up blood spills or spills of other potentially infectious material [1–3, 6, 11]:

1. Always wear protective gloves and any other personal protective equipment that might be appropriate for the situation. For example, if sharps (e.g., needles, syringes, or scalpels) are involved, use forceps to pick up the sharps and place the sharps in a puncture-resistant container.

2. When disinfecting, use an EPA-registered antimicrobial product that has specific claims against HIV or hepatitis B virus (which includes EPA-approved products) or use a freshly diluted sodium hypochlorite (bleach) solution. The bleach solution should be 1:100 for a small spill. If it is a large spill, use 1:10 dilution for the first application before cleaning (decontamination) and then use 1:100 for disinfection.

3. Clean the spill with disposable absorbent material and discard the contaminated materials into appropriate hazardous waste containers.

Special Situations

When an outbreak of *Clostridium difficile* is suspected or confirmed, special instructions for cleaning and disinfection need to be followed. This is because the organism produces spores that can live in the environment for many months, and these spores are highly resistant to cleaning and disinfection. During a suspected outbreak, first clean the objects using a diluted bleach solution (1:10 dilution or 1 part bleach to 9 parts water that is prepared daily). A diluted bleach solution is recommended because no EPA-registered disinfectant is specific for inactivating *Clostridium difficile* spores. Allow a contact time of 1 min by thoroughly wetting the surface with the diluted bleach solution and then allowing it to air-dry [13, 14].

When norovirus is suspected or confirmed, diluted bleach with a minimum concentration of 1:50 and a contact time of 1 min is recommended. However, bleach is substantially and quickly inactivated in the presence of organic matter. In areas with high levels of soiling and resistant surfaces, a 1:10 diluted bleach solution and a contact time of up to 10 min may be necessary. Because these concentrations are much higher than is allowed for a no-rinse food contact surface sanitizer according to the FDA Food Code, if the area is a food contact area, this disinfection procedure must be followed by a clear water rinse and a final wipe down with a sanitizing bleach solution of 1:200 to remove residual high levels

of bleach. Clean the area or objects (i.e., wash and scrub using a detergent), then disinfect the area [13, 14].

Eco-friendly and Nonchemical Alternatives

Successful green cleaning programs are gaining more acceptance in the cleaning process as nonchemical or less toxic alternatives by identifying new technologies, building materials, work practices (e.g., how cleaning products are used and disposed, how cleaning tasks are performed, or the physical conditions in which cleaning is performed) as a means of strengthening infection prevention and control goals. For example, microfiber mops and cloths have been shown as effective and safe alternatives to traditional rag mops, decreasing the use of harsh chemical cleaners, and potentially reducing back pain and injury from water buckets and mops. An entire building and its operational design needs to be considered for environmentally friendlier cleaning strategies. This may range from choosing surface materials that are easy to maintain and clean with the greenest product available to minimizing patient and worker exposure to cleaning and disinfecting products [14].

Biomedical Waste Management

The biomedical waste is the waste that is generated during the diagnosis, treatment, or immunization of human beings or animals or in research activities pertaining thereto, or in the production or testing of biological components [15, 16]. "Hospital waste" refers to all waste, biological or nonbiological, that is discarded and not intended for further use [17]. The waste produced in the course of health-care activities, from contaminated needles to radioactive isotopes, carries a greater potential for causing infection and injury than any other type of waste [18]. Hospital waste is a potential reservoir of microorganisms and requires safe and appropriate

Table 8.1 Categories of biomedical waste and color coding of waste bags

Waste category	Type of waste	Color coding	Treatment and disposal option
Category No. 1	Human anatomical waste (human tissues, organs, body parts)	Yellow	Incineration/deep burial
Category No. 2	Animal waste (animal tissues, organs, body parts, carcasses, bleeding parts, fluid, blood, and experimental animals used in research, waste generated by veterinary hospitals and colleges, discharge from hospitals, animal houses)	Yellow	Incineration/deep burial
Category No. 3	Microbiology and biotechnology waste (wastes from laboratory cultures, stocks or specimen of live microorganisms, or attenuated vaccines, human and animal cell cultures used in research and infectious agents from research and industrial laboratories, wastes from production of biologicals, toxins, and devices used for transfer of cultures)	Yellow, red	Local autoclaving/microwaving/incineration
Category No. 4	Waste sharps (needles, syringes, scalpels, blades, glass)	Blue/white Translucent plastic bag/puncture	Disinfecting (chemical treatment/autoclaving/microwaving and mutilation/shredding
Category No. 5	Discarded medicine and cytotoxic drugs (wastes comprising of outdated, contaminated, and discarded medicines)	Black	Incineration/destruction and drugs disposal in secured landfills
Category No. 6	Soiled waste (items contaminated with body fluids including cotton, dressings, soiled plaster casts, lines, bedding, and other materials contaminated with blood)	Yellow, red	Incineration/autoclaving/microwaving
Category No. 7	Solid waste (waste generated from disposable items other than the waste sharps such as tubing, catheters, intravenous sets)	Red, blue/white Translucent plastic bag/puncture	Disinfecting by chemical treatment/autoclaving/microwaving and mutilation/shredding
Category No. 8	Liquid waste (waste generated from the laboratory and washing, cleaning, housekeeping, and disinfecting activities)		Disinfecting by chemical Treatment and discharge into drains
Category No. 9	Incineration ash (ash from incineration of any biomedical waste)	Black	Disposal in municipal landfill
Category No. 10	Chemical waste (chemicals used in production of biological, chemicals used in disinfecting, as insecticides, etc.)	Black	Chemical treatment and discharge into drains for liquids and secured landfill for solids

handling and disposal. Its inadequate or inappropriate management may have serious public health consequences and deleterious effects on the environment. The most important and serious risk associated with hospital waste is sharps contaminated with blood/infectious body fluids. The waste as a whole generated from a hospital may not be more infectious than domestic waste. However, certain categories of waste (infected sharps, microbiological waste, chemical waste, and waste from certain contagious infections)

pose a high degree of health hazard, requiring special treatment. The biomedical wastes generated in the hospital are categorized as shown in Table 8.1 [16, 18].

The different location or points of generation of waste in a health-care establishment are:
1. Operation theatres/ICUs/wards/labor rooms
2. Dressing rooms
3. Injection rooms
4. Intensive care units
5. Dialysis room

6. Laboratories
7. Blood banks
8. Radio-diagnostic services
9. General hospital areas
10. Corridors
11. Compound of hospital or nursing home
12. Radiotherapy rooms
13. Canteen and kitchens
14. Laundry and CSSD

Biomedical Waste Management Rules 1998

The Biomedical Waste Management Rules were published on 20/07/1998 under Environment Protection Act 1986. As per this rule, every occupier of an institution generating biomedical waste, which includes hospitals, nursing home, clinic, dispensary, veterinary institutions, animal house, pathological laboratories, and blood banks, should take all steps to ensure that such a waste is handled without any adverse effect to human health and environment [15, 16].

Every occupier of an institution generating, collecting, receiving, storing, transporting, treating, disposing, and/or handling biomedical waste in any other manner, except such occupier of clinics, dispensaries, pathological laboratories, and blood banks providing treatment/service to less than 1,000 patient per month, is required to make an application to the prescribed authority for grant of authorization. Every operator of a biomedical waste facility is also required to make an application to the prescribed authority for grant of authorization. All biomedical waste has to be treated and disposed of in accordance with recommended procedures.

Waste Categories

Table 8.1 describes the categories of waste, the specified containers/bags for their collection, and the recommended treatment methodologies for hospital wastes [7, 10, 16, 18].

Handling of Waste

The organization and management of waste disposal requires a well-coordinated effort from hospital managers, infection control teams, nurses, sanitary staff, and all HCPs who are "generators" of the waste [10]. A waste management plan must be framed at national and local health regulatory level, based on the assessment of the current situation. Waste treatment can be done at a centralized facility or may be on site. The steps involved in the management of biomedical waste include waste generation, segregation, collection, transport, storage, treatment, and final disposal [10, 18, 19].

Every health-care facility should have a written document for waste handling, management, and transport, which should be regularly updated. All categories of health-care workers should be trained in handling waste and managing spillage [7, 10, 18]. They should be appropriately vaccinated and provided with PPE. All waste generated from the hospitals should be handled using standard precautions. Special care should be taken while handling and disinfecting/mutilating sharps.

The most essential element of biomedical waste management is segregation. This is because of two reasons:

1. Approximately 75–90 % of the biomedical waste is non-hazardous and harmless like any other municipal waste, the remaining being hazardous to humans/animals/aquatic life and deleterious to environment.
2. The hazardous waste requires special treatment, so that it is made harmless at the time of disposal. Since the different categories of hazardous waste require different treatment methods, it is important to segregate the hazardous waste in order to treat the waste appropriately.

Since the bulk of waste generated in hospitals is non-hazardous, it is of utmost importance to segregate the wastes so that treatment facilities can be optimally utilized. Segregation thus effectively improves the efficiency of treatment/disinfection procedures and ultimately reduces the cost of treatment. Inappropriate segregation results in mixing of hospital wastes with general waste, making the whole bulk of waste hazardous, which results in an incorrect method of waste disposal [7, 10, 15–20].

Segregation begins at the point of generation (source). It is the responsibility of the waste generator to segregate the waste at the point of generation. The waste should be segregated and discarded in specified, color-coded bags/containers, as shown in Table 8.1. These bags should be conveniently located, near the point of generation, and should be easily accessible. The waste bags should be of good quality and of suitable sizes for each patient care area. Instructions on waste separation should be posted at each waste collection point to remind the staff of the procedures. The color coding of the bags should also be taught to the staff on a regular basis. Staff should not attempt to correct errors of segregation by removing items from a bag or container after disposal or by placing one bag inside another bag of a different color. If general and hazardous wastes are accidentally mixed, the mixture should be treated as hazardous health-care waste [7, 10, 15–20]. The waste bags should be tied once they are filled ¾ of its capacity. The bags should not be closed by stapling. The health facilities should frame their own schedule for removal of waste in each shift or more frequently, depending on the amount of waste generated. All bags should be labeled with details of their point of production (hospital and ward or department) and contents. They should also be labeled with appropriate bio-hazard symbols. The bags or containers should be replaced immediately with new ones of the same type. A transfer note should include the description of waste being sent for disposal [7, 10, 18–20]. The collecting persons should ensure that the bags are properly labeled, tied and non-leaky. If the bags are torn or leaking, they should be placed in another bag of the same color-code.

Transport of biomedical waste bags: The waste bags being handed over for disposal should be counted and noted. Transport of waste is of two types: intramural (internal) and extra-mural (external). Intramural transport involves the movement of waste bags inside the health-care setup, whereas extramural transport involves their movement outside hospital for off-site treatment and/or disposal.

During intramural transport, separate trolleys should be used for transporting wastes (hazardous and non-hazardous). These trolleys should be cleaned and disinfected daily with an appropriate disinfectant. All waste bag seals should be in place and intact at the end of transportation [7, 10, 18–20]. Trash chutes should not be used for infectious/biomedical waste, since any accidentally torn bags would contaminate the entire chute. The waste routes must be designated to avoid passage of waste through patient care area.

For extramural movement, the HCF should ensure proper transport for off-site treatment. They are responsible for ensuring that a contractor is authorized to transport and dispose of waste. Any transport of untreated infectious/biomedical waste over public roads should follow federal rules and regulations [7, 10, 18–20].

The storage area for hospital waste should be in a secured hospital location, with limited access. It should be easy to clean, roofed, properly drained, and rodent and insect proof. Water supply for cleaning the facility is essential. There should be good lighting and passive ventilation. It should be preferably outside the immediate patient care facility and not be situated in the proximity of food stores or food preparation areas. A supply of cleaning equipment, protective clothing, and waste bags or containers should be located conveniently, close to the storage area. The area should be marked with a biohazard symbol [7, 10, 18–20]. All personnel entering the storage area should wear PPE.

Disposal and Treatment of Biomedical Waste

Various methods are used to treat and dispose of biomedical waste, including municipal dumping/deep burial, incineration, autoclaving, microwaving, and chemical disinfection. Special methods are required for handling cytotoxic and radioactive waste.

Municipal Dumping of General (Non-hazardous) Waste: Non-hazardous waste may be disposed of in municipal dumps. The municipal disposal may be in open dumps (which are not preferred) or sanitary landfills (preferred for hospital wastes). Only black bags are to be used for this purpose. The burial should be deep (2–3 m) and at least 1.5 m above ground water table [7, 10, 18].

Incineration: It is a high-temperature dry oxidation process, which results in a very significant reduction of waste volume and size. The most reliable and commonly used treatment process for health-care waste is pyrolytic incineration, also called controlled air incineration or double-chamber incineration [7, 10, 18]. The following types of waste are suitable for incineration: low heating value, above 2,000 kcal/kg (8,370 kJ/kg) for single-chamber incinerators and above 3,500 kcal/kg (14,640 kJ/kg) for pyrolytic double-chamber incinerators; content of combustible matter above 60 %; content of noncombustible solids below 5 %; content of noncombustible fines below 20 %; and moisture content below 30 %. Waste types which should not be incinerated include pressurized containers, halogenated plastics (PVC), high mercury or cadmium wastes, and ampoules containing heavy metals and glass. The ash produced in incinerators is sent for landfill.

Autoclaving: This is an efficient wet thermal disinfection process. It uses the principle of destruction of microorganism by steam under pressure. Highly infectious wastes should be preferably sterilized immediately by autoclaving. It therefore needs to be packaged in bags that are compatible with the proposed treatment process (blue/red plastic bags). The autoclaving cycle should at 121 °C for 15 min or 134 °C for 4 min. Since autoclaves are used in hospitals for the sterilization of reusable medical equipment, they allow for the treatment of only limited quantities of waste. Therefore, they are commonly used only for highly infectious waste, such as microbial cultures or sharps. It is recommended that all general hospitals, even those with limited resources, be equipped with autoclaves [7, 10, 18].

Microwave Irradiation: Most microorganisms are destroyed by the action of microwaves of a frequency of about 2,450 MHz and a wavelength of 12.24 cm. The water contained within the wastes is rapidly heated by the microwaves, and the infectious components are destroyed by heat conduction. In a microwave treatment unit, a loading device transfers the wastes into a shredder, where it is reduced to small pieces. The waste is then humidified, transferred to the irradiation chamber, which is equipped with a series of microwave generators, and irradiated for about 20 min. After irradiation, the waste is compacted inside a container and enters the municipal waste stream [18].

Chemical Disinfection: Chemical disinfection is now being used for the treatment of health-care waste. Chemicals are added to waste to kill or inactivate the pathogens [18]. This treatment usually results in disinfection rather than sterilization. Chemical disinfection is most suitable for treating liquid waste such as blood, urine, stools, or hospital sewage. However, solid and even highly hazardous health-care wastes, including microbiological cultures, sharps, etc., may also be disinfected chemically. This method has the following limitations: shredding and/or milling of waste is usually necessary before disinfection; powerful disinfectants are required, which are themselves also hazardous and should be used only by well trained and adequately protected personnel; disinfection efficiency depends on operational conditions; and only the surface of intact solid waste will be disinfected. Chemicals used for disinfection of health-care waste are mostly aldehydes, chlorine compounds, ammonium salts, and phenolic compounds.

Handling, Treatment, and Disposal of Sharps

Collection of Sharps: All sharps should be collected together, regardless of whether or not they are contaminated [7, 10, 18–20]. The containers for their collection should be puncture-proof (usually made of metal or high-density plastic) and fitted with covers. They should safely retain the sharps as well as any residual liquids from syringes. These containers should also be labeled with the biohazard symbol. To discourage misuse, containers should be tamper proof and needles and syringes should be rendered unusable [7, 10, 18–20].

Needles may be destroyed by the following methods:

1. By a needle destroying machine.
2. Remove needle by mechanically cutting tip of syringe, followed by sealing in metal container, smelting, or burying. The sharps may also be treated by plasma pyrolysis of puncture-proof containers storing the discarded sharps.

The syringes should be disinfected by either chemical treatment/autoclaving/microwaving. They may also be shredded in a shredder, followed by disposing in municipal dumps.

Handling and Treatment of Liquid Waste: Liquid biomedical waste is segregated and contained in leakproof, rigid containers. These containers are labeled with the biohazard symbol. Liquid waste is decontaminated at the site of generation with an approved chemical decontamination agent. If transport is required before decontamination, transport through public hallways should be kept to a minimum. The primary container must be placed within a secondary leakproof, rigid container (e.g., pail, box, or bin) during any transport. This secondary container must also be labeled with the biohazard symbol. Usually, the liquid waste is disinfected with 1 % sodium hypochlorite and discharged into drains/sewers (dilution and disposal). However, excessive use of chemical disinfectants should be avoided as it may be a health and environmental hazard [7, 10, 18–20].

Treatment of Radioactive and Cytotoxic Waste: Special facilities are required for radioactive and cytotoxic materials and pharmaceutical chemicals. These wastes must be handled in accordance with federal and state regulations.

References

1. Guidelines for Environmental Infection Control in Health-Care Facilities. Recommendations of CDC and the Healthcare Infection Control Practices Advisory Committee (HICPAC). U.S. Department of Health and Human Services, Centers for Disease Control and Prevention. 2003.
2. Infection control guidelines. Communicable disease report, Laboratory Centre for Disease Control Bureau of Infectious Diseases, Canada. 1998.
3. Rutala WA, Weber DJ. Disinfection and sterilization in health care facilities: what clinicians need to know. Clin1 Infect Dis. 2004;39:702–9.
4. Ruden H, Daschner F. Should we routinely disinfect floors? J Hosp Infect. 2002;51:309.
5. Rutala WA, Weber DJ. The benefits of surface disinfection. Am J Infect Control. 2004;32:226–31.
6. Rutala WA, Weber DJ, The Healthcare Infection Control Practices Advisory Committee (HICPAC). Guideline for disinfection and sterilization in healthcare facilities. Washington, DC: Centers for Disease control and Prevention; 2008.
7. Ayeliff GAJ, Fraise AP, Geddes AM, Mitchell K. Control of hospital infection. 4th ed. New York: Arnold; 2000.
8. Dharan S, Mourouga P, Copin P, et al. Routine disinfection of patients' environmental surfaces. Myth or reality? J Hosp Infect. 1999;42:113–17.
9. Maki DG, Alvarado CJ, Hassemer CA, Zilz MA. Relation of the inanimate hospital environment to endemic nosocomial infection. N Engl J Med. 1982;307:1562–6.
10. World Health Organization. Guidelines on prevention and control of hospital associated infections. South East Asian Region: WHO; 2002.
11. Infection control guidelines for the prevention of transmission of infectious diseases in the health care setting. Communicable Diseases Network Australia, the National Public Health Partnership and the Australian Health, Ministers' Advisory Council, January 2004.
12. http://www.ems.org.eg/esic_home/data/gived_part1/ceaning.pdf
13. www.education.nh.gov/instruction/school_health/documents/disinfectant.pdf
14. Pia Markkanen, Margaret Quinn, Catherine Galligan, Anila Bello. Cleaning in healthcare facilities. Reducing human health effects and environmental impacts. Health care research collaborative. April 2009. http://www.sustainableproduction.org/downloads/CleaninginHealthcareFacilities.pdf
15. Razdan P, Cheema AS. Bio-medical waste management system. http://220.156.188.21/CDAC/ASCNT_2009/ASCNT%202009/Paper/HIS/Abstract26.pdf
16. Govt of India, Ministry of Environment and Forests Gazette notification No 460 dated July 27, New Delhi. 1998:10–20. http://envfor.nic.in/legis/hsm/biomed.html
17. Rutala WA. Medical waste. Infect Control Hosp Epidemiol. 1992;13(1):38–48.
18. Pruss A, Giroult E, Rushbrook P. Safe management of waste from health care activities. http://www.who.int/water_sanitation_health/medicalwaste/wastemanag/en/
19. Biomedical Waste Disposal Procedures. http://www.uottawa.ca/services/ehss/biosafety.htm
20. Infectious/Biomedical Waste Management Plan. www.ehs.washington.edu

Part VII

Hand Hygiene and Personal Protective Equipment

Hand Hygiene and Personal Protective Equipment

9

Arti Kapil

Healthcare-associated infections (HAIs) are responsible for increase in morbidity and mortality in hospitalized patients in developing countries [1]. These infections add to the cost of the already burdened healthcare settings in resource-limited countries, and strategies to control them need to be cost-effective and evidence based. Hand hygiene has been considered as a single most important intervention to reduce preventable HAIs in the resource-poor countries [2]. Hand hygiene has been an important cultural practice in India. Though in ancient times the mode of transmission of disease through hands was not scientifically proven, contaminated hands were associated with unhygienic practices leading to illness. Semmelweiss in the nineteenth century showed that use of clean hands for conducting delivery reduced the maternal mortality rate, which was further evidenced through research that hand antisepsis reduces the transmission of pathogens and the incidence of HAIs [2, 3].

Role of Hand Hygiene in Transmission of Infections

There has been enough evidence that the hands of the healthcare workers are the most common vehicle for the transmission of healthcare-associated pathogens from patient to patient and within the healthcare environment and studies show a direct correlation of increase adherence to hand hygiene and decrease in HAIs [4]. It not only reduces cross infection in the hospitals; it also is an integral part of standard precautions and practice of use of personal protective equipment for safety of healthcare workers [5].

Even in the community level, the association of hand hygiene and decrease in infection has been supported by evidence base. In a recently published meta-analysis, the strength of the association as measured by the relative reduction in risk of illness was appreciable with practice of hand hygiene, and the evidence suggests that personal and environmental hygiene reduces the spread of infection [6].

World Health Organization Initiative and Definitions

This evidence prompted the WHO to bring out guidelines on the practice of hand hygiene in 2009 [7]. In addition, the main objective of the First Global Patient Safety Challenge launched by the World Health Organization was to achieve an improvement in hand hygiene practices worldwide with the ultimate goal of promoting a strong patient safety culture.

A. Kapil, M.D. (✉)
Department of Microbiology, AIIMS,
New Delhi, India
e-mail: akapilmicro@gmail.com

C. Wattal and N. Khardori (eds.), *Hospital Infection Prevention: Principles & Practices*,
DOI 10.1007/978-81-322-1608-7_9, © Springer India 2014

WHO has Defined Certain Terms in Relation to Hand Hygiene

1. *Antiseptic hand washing.* Washing hands with soap and water or other detergents containing an antiseptic agent.
2. *Antiseptic hand rubbing (or hand rubbing).* Applying an antiseptic hand rub to reduce or inhibit the growth of microorganisms without the need for an exogenous source of water and requiring no rinsing or drying with towels or other devices.
3. *Hand antisepsis/decontamination/degerming.* Reducing or inhibiting the growth of microorganisms by the application of an antiseptic hand rub or by performing an antiseptic hand wash.
4. *Patient zone.* Concept related to the "geographical" visualization of key moments for hand hygiene. It contains the patient X and his/her immediate surroundings. This typically includes the intact skin of the patient and all inanimate surfaces that are touched by or in direct physical contact with the patient such as the bed rails, bedside table, bed linen, infusion tubing, and other medical equipment. It further contains surfaces frequently touched by HCWs while caring for the patient such as monitors, knobs, and buttons and other "high-frequency" touch surfaces.
5. *Healthcare area* The *healthcare area* corresponds to all surfaces in the healthcare setting outside the patient zone of patient X, i.e., other patients and their patient zones and the wider healthcare environment.
6. *Point of care.* The place where three elements come together: the patient, the HCW, and care or treatment involving contact with the patient or his/her surroundings (within the patient zone). The concept embraces the need to perform hand hygiene at recommended moments exactly where care delivery takes place. This requires that a hand hygiene product (e.g., alcohol-based hand rub, if available) be easily accessible and as close as possible – within arm's reach – of where patient care or treatment is taking place.

Point-of-care products should be accessible without having to leave the patient zone.

Dynamics of Transmission of Pathogens by Hands

To understand the mode of transmission through hands and plan intervention, it is important to understand the dynamics of the transmission of infection via hands.

Types of Bacterial Flora of Hand
The hands can carry two types of bacterial flora:
1. *Resident flora* – This is a part of the normal flora of hands and has negligible pathogenic potential. If introduced into the sterile sites during trauma or any invasive procedure, it can cause infection. This cannot be easily removed by hand washing.
2. *Transient flora* – These are carried on the hands that get contaminated in the healthcare setting due to handling of patients, equipment, or environment. They are responsible for cross infection in settings and are easily removed by hand hygiene.

Transmission Cycle
For a successful transmission of pathogens from one patient to another via HCW hands, five sequential steps are required to complete the transmission cycle:
 (i) Bacteria should be present on the patient's skin or inanimate objects in the surrounding.
 (ii) Bacteria must be transferred to the hands of HCWs.
 (iii) Bacteria survive for some time on the hands.
 (iv) Hand hygiene by the HCW must be inappropriate either absent or by virtue of wrong method or wrong agent.
 (v) The contaminated hands must come into direct contact with another patient or with an inanimate object which can come in direct contact with the patient.

Figure 9.1 shows how contaminated hands can transfer bacteria within and outside a healthcare setting.

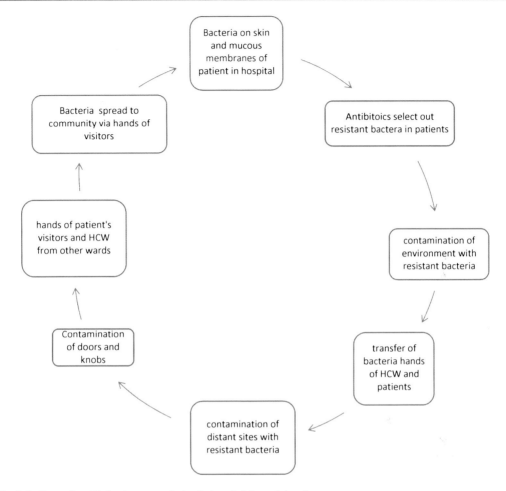

Fig. 9.1 Dynamics of infection transmission in hospital through hands

Infrastructure Required for Practice of Hand Hygiene

The kind of infrastructure and material required to practice hand hygiene will depend on whether soap and water or alcohol-based method is to be practiced.

Hand Wash

The facilities required are a tap with safe water source and sink, liquid soap with dispenser, and a disposable sterile towel. Hand wash with soap and water acts by removal of bacteria and other organic material from hand. Addition of antibacterial agent improves the efficacy significantly rather than plain soap.

Hand Rub

Alcohol-based hand rub with 60–80 % alcohol requires a dispensable bottle, preferably wall mounted at the bedside. Only ensure that the hands must be completely wet with the hand rub at the time of application. The main advantage is that alcohol-based hand rubs do not need water which may not be easily available at each place and with continuous supply. The safe water is another restriction in the resource-limited countries. Sterile towels are expensive. The presence of alcohol-based hand rubs in the point of care improves hand hygiene compliance and helps in the sustenance of the practice [8, 9]. Addition of emollients helps in reducing skin dryness and irritation.

The greatest challenge for the use of alcohol-based hand rubs has remained their ineffectiveness on the *Clostridium difficile* spores. It has been a cause of worry that the use of alcohol-based hand rubs may select out *C. difficile* spores in a hospital environment. Though a possibility exists theoretically, the temporal association has not been shown between the two. To determine the selection of *C. difficile* spores on hands after using the alcohol-based hand rub, a study was carried out on the volunteers. It was found that the colony count of *C. difficile* on the inoculated hands of volunteers did not show any reduction after alcohol-based hand rubs, whereas with soap and water, there was a reduction. Further the transmissibility of these spores by contact was also determined and it was shown that the transfer from hand to hand was also efficient [10, 11]. Though direct evidence of CDI disease and use of alcohol-based hand is not there, till such time that this resolves, it is advisable to use soap and water in settings where CD contamination is known [12].

Compliance

Although hand hygiene is the leading measure for reducing healthcare-associated infections, healthcare worker compliance remains low in most settings due to various factors. Many reasons have been mentioned by the different workers including lack of time and resources, emergency situations, or irritation to skin [2, 4]. However, it is observed that mainly the attitude and behavioral change is required for successful implementation of hand hygiene practices in the healthcare settings [13].

Perception of Infection Control Practices – The lack of education and understanding of the risk of acquisition of infection are some of the other factors which must be addressed. Ongoing education is an important component which may increase adherence of the practices.

Job and professional qualification has been observed to be one of the risk factors involved with hand hygiene [14, 15]. We carried out a study to assess the existing level of knowledge, attitudes, and practices towards infection control among resident doctors and nurses of a tertiary care hospital by means of a Knowledge Attitude Practices (KAP) questionnaire, which had a strong component on hand hygiene and its role in reducing healthcare-associated infections. Although the mean total score among doctors and nurses showed no statistically significant difference, the doctors had significantly higher scores than nurses in the knowledge and attitude components, whereas nurses had scored significantly higher in the practice component [16].

Implementation

Implementation of the hand hygiene guidelines remains a challenge. A review of the Cochrane Database Review System on the subject has revealed that the quality of intervention studies intended to increase hand hygiene compliance remains disappointing [17]. Although campaigns with social marketing or involvement of the staff seem to have an effect, there is an insufficient evidence to draw a firm conclusion. There remains an urgent need to undertake research to explore the effectiveness of properly designed and implemented interventions to increase hand hygiene compliance so as to convince the doctors, nurses, and other support staff. As per the document of WHO Implementation of the Multimodal Hand Hygiene Improvement Strategy [7], there are five strategies to improve/implement hand hygiene practices in a healthcare organization, which can be initiated in a healthcare setting so as to understand specific needs, identify lacunae, and accordingly improve the practices.

The effectiveness of WHO strategy has been tested in some settings and found useful.

Some of the recently published intervention studies in long-term care facility in a hospital determined the multimodal strategy in promoting hand hygiene in a cluster randomized controlled trial which showed a significant increase in compliance after intervention [18]. At that time, the outbreaks of respiratory tract infections and MRSA infections requiring hospital admission were reduced after intervention. Similarly, a multifaceted hand hygiene involving use of pocket-sized containers of antiseptic gel also showed a significant increase in compliance to hand hygiene as compared to control groups. The incident of serious infections decreased along with pneumonia, and death rate due to infections decreased in the intervention group in a clustered randomized controlled trial done in a long-term care facility [8].

Hand Hygiene and Control of Antimicrobial Resistance

The systematic review of well-designed studies shows that hand hygiene has also contributed to the control of antimicrobial resistance indirectly by reducing the transmission of infections and reducing colonization of mucosal surfaces. This would therefore decrease the use of antibiotics, thus reducing antibiotic selective pressure [19].

Systems-level efforts to implement the guidelines were associated with lower rates of MRSA and VRE. Significant reduction in rates of resistance among *Klebsiella* isolates occurred after an intervention that included emphasis on hand hygiene, gloves, and education about the use of antibiotics [20, 21].

To explore the dynamics of MDRO transmission in the hospital, a model was developed extending data from clinical individual-level studies to quantify the impact of hand hygiene, contact precautions, reducing antimicrobial exposure, and screening surveillance cultures in decreasing the prevalence of MDRO colonization and infection. Hand hygiene had the most beneficial effect, as it limits transmission from all colonized patients, including those who are known and unknown to be colonized [22]. Various steps to hand washing are shown in Fig. 9.2 [7]. Various concentrations of disinfectants have been explained in Fig. 9.3.

Six Steps of hand washing

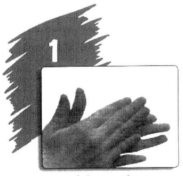

Palm to palm

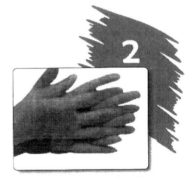

Palm to palm, interlaced

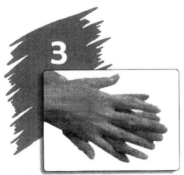

Right palm over left dorsum and
left palm over right dorsum

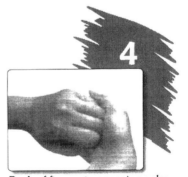

Back of fingers to opposing palm
with fingers interlocked

Fig. 9.2 Six steps of hand washing [7]

Work into left thumb with right hand.
Change hands and repeat

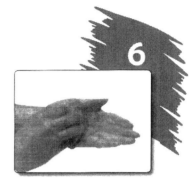

Right hand fingertips into palm of hand.
Change hands and repeat.

Fig. 9.2 (continued)

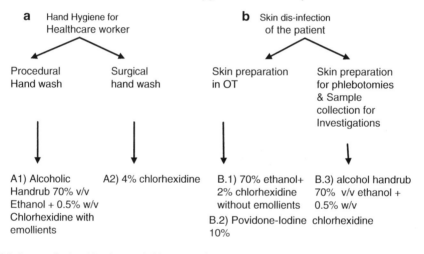

Fig. 9.3 Disinfectants for hand hygiene and skin preparation

Personal Protective Equipment

PPE provides a physical barrier to prevent direct contact of the HCW with infectious material [5]. The contact could be (a) with the hands, eyes, clothes, or any other part of the body or (b) between patients.

The types of PPE are gloves, goggles, mask, apron, gown, boots or shoe cover, and cap (Table 9.1). The use of PPE would depend on exposure expected but gloves remain constant as a part of standard precautions.

The PPE should be worn not only by HCW taking care of patients but also by support staff who may handle contaminated material while cleaning, laboratory personnel, and family parents who are in contact with gloves from all important additional component of hand hygiene as well as personal protective equipment. They are integral part of standard precautions that must be practiced irrespective of the infectious status of the patient. Gloves must be worn when handling excretions or secretions that may or may not be contaminated with blood.

Table 9.1 Indications of use of personal protective equipment[a]

Gloves	Mask	Eye wear goggles/shield	Caps/boot/shoe cover	Gown/apron
Nonsterile/clean Touching body fluids	Wear when exposure expected over the face	When procedures generating splashes	When splash may contaminate hair, shoes, etc.	Use impermeable gowns
Change between patient	Avoid use of cotton or gauge masks			Protect skin/clothes etc. during splash generating procedure
Change between tasks on same patient	N-95 mask is used for protection of health workers			
Wash hands after removal of gloves				
Dispose used gloves and do not reuse				
Sterile gloves – for aseptic procedures				

[a]Dispose all the PPE as per the waste handling rules

Education and training is an important component in order to effectively use PPE.

Discard all the above as per waste handling rules.

Order/Sequence of Donning PPE

Wearing – The order of PPE should be followed. The order of PPE to be followed should be gown first, mask, goggles, and gloves.

Removal – Gloves, goggle, gown, and mask.

Precautions – Do not touch face or adjust PPE surfaces after wearing gloves. Remove gloves if torn and wash hands before wearing fresh gloves.

Conclusions

Hand hygiene remains a single most cost-effective hospital infection control measure. It is also an integral component of standard precautions and, specifically, targeted "isolation precautions" (namely, contact, droplet, and airborne precautions). It is also emphasized in all the "bundle care" approaches for the prevention of infections such as device-related infections, bloodstream infections, urinary tract infections, surgical site infection, and ventilator-associated pneumonia. Alcohol-based hand rubs should be encouraged as chances of compliance increase due to its easy availability at the point of care. In situations where residual activity is necessary, chlorhexidine-based formulations can be used. However, if the hands are visibly soiled, or during enteric precautions, hand washing with antimicrobial soap and water is mandatory.

Systems approach and commitment from management is important for effective practice of hand hygiene in a healthcare setting. The policy must address the availability of primary facilities, training, and implementation of hand hygiene practices. The hospitals must carry out their own studies so that they understand lacunae in the practices of hand hygiene. Ensuring compliance is a big challenge and there is a need for regular monitoring of compliance so as to identify decline of compliance followed by corrective action and continual improvement.

Channelizing the resources towards provision of facilities for appropriate hand hygiene and continuous education of healthcare personnel, and population in general, is a cost-effective method to decrease the HAIs and antibiotic resistance.

References

1. Gupta A, Kapil A, Lodha R, Kabra SK, Sood S, Dhawan B, Das BK, Sreenivas V. Burden of healthcare-associated infections in a paediatric intensive care unit of a developing country: a single centre experience using active surveillance. J Hosp Infect. 2011;78(4):323–6.

2. Allegranzi B, Pittet D. Role of hand hygiene in healthcare-associated infection prevention. J Hosp Infect. 2009;73:305–15.

3. Rosenthal VD, Guzman S, Safdar N. Reduction in nosocomial infection with improved hand hygiene in intensive care units of a tertiary care hospital in Argentina. Am J Infect Control. 2000;28:3.

4. Pittet D. Improving compliance with hand hygiene in hospitals. Infect Control Hosp Epidemiol. 2000;21(6):381–6.

5. Siegel JD, Rhinehart E, Jackson M, Chiarello L. Preventing transmission of infectious agents in health-care settings. 2007. http://www.cdc.gov/ncidod/dhqp/pdf/isolation2007

6. Aiello AE, Larson EL. What is the evidence for a causal link between hygiene and infections? S Lancet Infect Dis. 2002;2:103–10.

7. WHO Guidelines on Hand Hygiene in Health Care. World Health Organization. 2009. www.who.int/publications/2009

8. Wing Kin Yeung, Wai San Wilson Tam, Tze Wai Wong. Clustered Randomized Controlled Trial of a Hand Hygiene Intervention Involving Pocket-Sized Containers of Alcohol-Based Hand Rub for the Control of Infections in Long-Term Care Facilities. Infect Control Hosp Epidemiol 2011;32(1):67–76.

9. Rupp ME, Fitzgerald T, Puumala S, et al. Prospective, controlled, crossover trial of alcohol-based hand gel in critical care units. Infect Control Hosp Epidemiol. 2008;29(1):8–15.

10. Jabbar EU, Leischner J, Kasper D, Gerber R, Sambol SP. Effectiveness of alcohol-based hand rubs for removal of *Clostridium difficile* from hands. Infect Control Hosp Epidemiol. 2010;31(6):565–70.

11. Boyce JM F, Ligi C, Kohan C, Dumigan D, Havill NL. Lack of association between the increased incidence of *Clostridium difficile*-associated disease and the increasing use of alcohol-based hand rubs. Infect Control Hosp Epidemiol. 2006;27(5):479–83.

12. Oughton MT, Loo VG, Dendukuri N, Fenn S, Libman MD. Hand hygiene with soap and water is superior to alcohol rub and antiseptic wipes for removal of *Clostridium difficile*. Infect Control Hosp Epidemiol. 2009;30:939–44.

13. Pitter D, Simon A, Hugonnet S, Pessoa-Silva CL, Sauvan V. Hand hygiene among physicians: performance, beliefs, and perceptions. Ann Intern Med. 2004;141:1–8.

14. Longtin Yves, Sax Hugo, Allegranzi Benedetta, Schneider Franck, Pitter Didier. Hand hygiene. N Engl J Med. 2011;364:e24.

15. Ashraf MS, Hussain SW, Agarwal N, Ashraf S, EL-Kass G. Hand hygiene in long-term care facilities: a multicenter study of knowledge, attitudes, practices, and barriers. Infect Control Hosp Epidemiol. 2010;31(7):758–62.

16. Gupta A, Kapil A, Lodha R, Sreenivas V. Knowledge, attitudes & practices towards infection control amongst the healthcare professionals. Natl Med J India. 2013;26:35–36.

17. Gould DJ, Moralejo D, Drey N, Chudleigh JH. Interventions to improve hand hygiene compliance in patient care. Cochrane Database Syst Rev. 2010;9, CD005186.

18. Mei-lin Ho, Wing-hong Seto, Lai-chin Wong, Tin-yau Wong. Effectiveness of Multifaceted Hand Hygiene Interventions in Long-Term Care Facilities in Hong Kong: A Cluster-Randomized Controlled Trial. Infect Control Hosp Epidemiol 2012;33(8):761–67

19. Siegel JD, Rhinehart E, Jackson M, Chiarello L. Management of multidrug-resistant organisms in healthcare settings. 2006. www.cdc.gov/hicpac/pdf/MDRO/MDROGuidline2006

20. Larson EL, RN, Quiros D, Giblin T, RN, Lin S. Relationship of antimicrobial control policies and hospital infection control characteristics to antimicrobial resistance rates. Am J Crit Care. 2007;16:110–20.

21. Aboelela SW, Saiman L, Stone P, Lowy FD, Quiros D, Larson E. Effectiveness of barrier precautions and surveillance cultures to control transmission of multidrug-resistant organisms: a systematic review of the literature. Am J Infect Control. 2006;34:484–94.

22. Wilton P, Smith R, Coast J, Millar M. Strategies to contain the emergence of antimicrobial resistance: a systematic review of effectiveness and cost-effectiveness. J Health Serv Res Policy. 2002;7(2):111–17.

Part VIII

Decontamination and Sterilization Procedures

Decontamination and Sterilization Procedures

10

Chand Wattal and J.K. Oberoi

The optimization of disinfection and sterilization procedures is important in preventing healthcare-associated infections. Data from the National Survey of Ambulatory Surgery (NSAS) showed that an estimated 53.3 million surgical and nonsurgical procedures were performed in the United States in 2006, including 9.2 million gastrointestinal endoscopies [1]. The introduction of pathogens leading to infection is the most common form of postoperative morbidity and a major cause of mortality in all such procedures. Disinfection and sterilization are essential to ensure that equipments and instruments used on patients do not transmit infections to them. Many outbreaks have been reported due to serious deficiencies in the disinfection and sterilization techniques employed in hospitals [2–4]. The goals of effective disinfection and sterilization of medical equipment/devices are, therefore, to prevent transmission of microorganisms to patients and hospital personnel and to minimize damage to medical equipment/devices from human material (e.g., blood, body fluids, saline, and medications) or inappropriate handling.

Definitions [5]

Sterilization refers to a physical or chemical process that completely destroys or removes all forms of viable microorganisms from an object, including spores. However, prions are not susceptible to routine sterilization. Sterility is an absolute condition – an item is either sterile or not sterile; there can be no thing as "partially sterile."

Cleaning is the removal of visible soil (e.g., organic and inorganic material) from objects and surfaces and is accomplished manually or mechanically using water with detergents or enzymatic products. Thorough cleaning is essential before high-level disinfection and/or sterilization because inorganic and organic materials that remain on the surfaces of instruments interfere with the effectiveness of these processes.

Disinfection or *decontamination* describes a process that eliminates many or all pathogenic microorganisms on inanimate objects, with the exception of bacterial spores to render objects safe to handle, use, or discard.

A *germicide* is an agent that can kill microorganisms, particularly pathogenic organisms ("germs"). The term *germicide* includes both antiseptics and disinfectants. *Antiseptics* are germicides applied to the living tissue and skin; *disinfectants* are antimicrobials only for inanimate objects.

C. Wattal, M.D. (✉) • J.K. Oberoi, M.D.
Department of Clinical Microbiology,
Sir Ganga Ram Hospital, New Delhi, India
e-mail: chandwattal@gmail.com

C. Wattal and N. Khardori (eds.), *Hospital Infection Prevention: Principles & Practices*,
DOI 10.1007/978-81-322-1608-7_10, © Springer India 2014

Spaulding's Classification

In 1968, Earle Spaulding devised a rational approach to disinfection and sterilization [6]. This is now referred to as Spaulding's classification and it has been refined and retained over the years. He described three categories: critical, semi-critical, and noncritical. According to Spaulding, the process and products used for disinfection and/or sterilization of medical equipment/devices depends on the intended use of the equipment/device and the potential risk of infection involved in the use of the equipment/device (Table 10.1).

Factors that affect both disinfection and sterilization include [5] the following:

- Prior cleaning of the object
- Organic and inorganic load present
- The number and level of microorganisms present on items to be disinfected
- Concentration of and exposure time to the germicide
- Effective contact between the biocidal agent and the microorganisms: structure of the equipment (presence of crevices, lumens, hinges) and biofilms
- Temperature and pH of the disinfection process and, in some cases, relative humidity of the sterilization process (e.g., ethylene oxide)

Cleaning

It is the removal of organic matter and microorganisms from a surface by a process such as washing with detergent without prior processing. Organic matter can interfere with the action of disinfectants on the microorganisms present on the surface of the devices to be sterilized. In addition, cleaning reduces the number of organisms to a minimum before exposing the equipment to the sterilizing or disinfecting process. An item that has not been adequately cleaned cannot be effectively disinfected or sterilized.

Cleaning may be done manually or mechanically (e.g., washer-disinfector, ultrasonic washer, washer-sterilizer) after gross soil has been removed. The two important features necessary for manual cleaning include friction and fluidics [5]. Friction (e.g., rubbing/scrubbing the soiled area with a brush) is universally used and for devices with small lumens where the brush cannot reach, fluidics (i.e., fluids under pressure) is used to remove soil and debris from internal channels after brushing. Gross soil should first be removed by rinsing with water, a detergent solution, or a detergent/disinfectant formulation immediately at point of use. Once medical equipment/devices have been received in the reprocessing area/department, they must be disassembled, sorted, and soaked. Soaking in an

Table 10.1 Spaulding's Classification [6] of medical equipment/devices and required level of processing/reprocessing

Classification	Definition	Level of processing/reprocessing	Examples
Critical equipment/ device	Equipment/device that enters sterile tissues, including the vascular system	Sterilization by steam, gas, hydrogen peroxide plasma, or chemical sterilants	Surgical instruments
			Cardiac catheters
			Implants
Semicritical equipment/device	Equipment/device that comes in contact with non- intact skin or mucous membranes but do not penetrate them	High-level disinfection (as a minimum): exposure time ≥12–30 min at 20 °C, sterilization is preferred	Respiratory therapy equipment
			Anesthesia equipment GI endoscopes
			Tonomoter
Noncritical equipment/device	Equipment/device that touches only intact skin and not mucous membranes, or does not directly touch the client/patient/resident	Low-level disinfection: exposure time: ≥1 min or detergent cleaning	ECG machines
			Oximeters
			Bedpans, urinals, commodes

enzymatic solution may be required if the exudate has dried [7, 8]. Neutral or near-neutral pH detergent solutions are preferred for cleaning as these are generally compatible with instrument materials and also lead to good soil removal. Enzymes, mainly proteases, can also be added to detergents as these aid in the removal of organic matter but need to be finally rinsed off the instruments to prevent adverse chemical reactions [9]. Although the effectiveness of high-level disinfection and sterilization mandates effective cleaning, no "real-time" tests exist that can be employed in a clinical setting to verify cleaning. At a minimum, all instruments should be individually inspected and be visibly clean.

Disinfection

The effective use of disinfectants is part of a multiple barrier strategy to prevent healthcare-associated infections. It may involve chemical or thermal means. Thermal disinfection is always preferable to chemical disinfection, provided the items can withstand it. A few disinfectants will kill spores with prolonged exposure times (3–12 h); these are called *chemical sterilants*. High-level disinfectants are chemical sterilants, which, when used for a shorter exposure period than would be required for sterilization, kill all microorganisms with the exception of a high number of bacterial spores. Intermediate-level disinfectants may kill mycobacteria, vegetative bacteria, most viruses, and most fungi but do not necessarily kill bacterial spores. Low-level disinfectants may kill most vegetative bacteria, some fungi, and some viruses within ≤10 min [5].

Chemical Disinfectants: A chemical disinfectant is a compound or mixture which, under defined conditions, is capable of destroying microorganisms by chemical or physicochemical means. It is usually in the form of a liquid and occasionally a gas. Disinfectants can be supplied ready to use or may need accurate dilution to appropriate in-use strength. Disinfectants vary in their properties (are not interchangeable), mak-

ing the correct choice of a disinfectant for a specific task in a particular set of circumstances important. Tables 10.2 and 10.3 give a detailed description of commonly available *high-level* and *low-level disinfectants*, respectively.

Thermal disinfection: It achieves high-level disinfection when surfaces are in contact with heated water for an appropriate length of time. It includes pasteurization and use of flushing and washer-disinfectors:

(A) Pasteurization: The time-temperature relation for hot-water pasteurization is generally ~70 °C (158 °F) for 30 min. Pasteurization of respiratory therapy and anesthesia equipment is a recognized alternative to chemical disinfection. Monitoring of the water temperature is important as part of a quality assurance program.

(B) Flushing and washer-disinfectors are automated and closed equipment that clean and disinfect objects like bedpans and washbowls, surgical instruments, and anesthesia tubes. A typical washer-disinfector cycle includes the following stages:
- Cold-water rinse
- Warm-water wash, with cleaning agent
- Hot-water rinse, with disinfection (e.g., 80–85 °C for 2 min or other intended conditions)
- Drying by radiant heat or hot air

Reprocessing of Endoscopes

A large number of healthcare-associated outbreaks have been linked to contaminated endoscopes than to any other medical device [10, 11]. Endoscopes are sophisticated, reusable instruments that have specific need to be cleaned, disinfected, and sterilized. According to the classification system proposed by DR EH Spaulding, endoscopes fall into the category of semi-critical items and receive, at a minimum, high-level disinfection after each use. This standard has been recommended by federal agencies such as the CDC and FDA [5, 12] as well as other professional

Table 10.2 High-level disinfectants (HLDs)

S. no.	Disinfectant	Mode of action	Microbicidal activity	Contact period	Uses	Monitoring	Advantages/comments	Disadvantages/comments
1	Glutaraldehyde 2 %	Alkylation of sulfhydryl, hydroxyl, carboxyl, and amino groups of microorganisms, leading to alteration of RNA, DNA, and protein synthesis	Spores+ Mycobacteria+ Bacteria+ Viruses+	HLD: 20–90 min at 20°–25 °C, sterilization 10 h at 20°–25 °C	Heat-sensitive equipment/devices, lensed instruments that do not require sterilization, endoscopes, respiratory therapy equipment, Anesthesia equipment	Exposure time and temperature must be maintained, test strips for concentration are available from the manufacturer and must be used at least daily (preferably with each load)	Relatively inexpensive, excellent materials compatibility, active in presence of organic material	Activation required, shelf life 14 days, respiratory irritation from glutaraldehyde, vapor, pungent and irritating odor, relatively slow mycobactericidal activity. Coagulates blood and fixes tissue to surfaces, allergic contact dermatitis. Glutaraldehyde vapor monitoring recommended
2	Accelerated hydrogen peroxide 7 %	Producing destructive hydroxyl free radicals that can attack membrane lipids, DNA, and other essential cell components	Spores+ Mycobacteria+ Bacteria+ Viruses+	HLD:30 min at 20°–25 °C, sterilization 6 h at 20°–25 °C	Heat-sensitive equipment/devices	Test kits to monitor the concentration are available from the manufacturer and must be used with each load	No activation required, may enhance removal of organic matter and organisms. No disposal issues. No odor or irritation issues. Does not coagulate blood or fix tissues to surfaces. Inactivates cryptosporidium	Material compatibility concerns (brass, zinc, copper, and nickel/silver plating) both cosmetic and functional. Serious eye damage with contact
3	Ortho-phthalaldehyde (OPA) (0.55 %)	Interact with amino acids, proteins, and microorganisms, kills spores by blocking the spore germination process	Spores+ Mycobacteria+ Bacteria+ Viruses+	HLD:12 min at 20° & 5 min at 25 °C, sterilization: no claim	Endoscopy equipment/devices (contraindicated for cystoscopes) Heat-sensitive equipment/devices	Test strips for concentration are available from the manufacturer and must be used at least daily (preferably with each load)	Fast acting high-level disinfectant, no activation required. Odor not significant, excellent materials compatibility claimed. Does not coagulate blood or fix tissues to surfaces claimed	Stains skin, mucous membranes, clothing, and environmental surfaces. Repeated exposure may result in hypersensitivity in some patients with bladder cancer. More expensive than glutaraldehyde. Eye irritation with contact. Slow sporicidal activity

Table 10.3 Low-level disinfectants

S. no.	Disinfectant	Mode of action	Microbicidal activity	Uses	Monitoring	Advantages/comments	Disadvantages/comments
1	Alcohols (60–95 %)	Denaturation of proteins	Spores − Mycobacteria + Bacteria + Viruses +	External surfaces of some equipment(e.g., stethoscopes, oral and rectal thermometers, ventilators, etc.) skin antiseptic	Not required	Nontoxic, cheap, rapid action, non-staining, no residue, effective on clean equipment/devices that can be immersed	Evaporates quickly – not a good surface disinfectant; flammable; coagulates protein; a poor cleaner; may dissolve lens mountings inactivated by organic material
2	Chlorines and chlorine compounds	Oxidation of sulfhydryl enzymes and amino acids; ring chlorination of amino acids; loss of intracellular contents; decreased uptake of nutrients; inhibition of protein synthesis; decreased oxygen uptake; oxidation of respiratory components; decreased adenosine triphosphate production; breaks in DNA; and depressed DNA synthesis	Spores + Mycobacteria + Bacteria + Viruses+	Hydrotherapy tanks, exterior surfaces of dialysis equipment, cardiopulmonary training manikins, environmental surface, noncritical equipment used for home healthcare, blood spills	Not required	Broad-spectrum, economical, fast acting	Corrosive to metals inactivated by organic material; for large blood spills, blood must be removed prior to disinfection; irritant to skin and mucous membranes; should be used immediately once diluted; use in well-ventilated areas; must be stored in closed containers away from ultraviolet light and heat to prevent deterioration
3	Accelerated hydrogen peroxide 0.5–3 %	Producing destructive hydroxyl free radicals that can attack membrane lipids, DNA, and other essential cell components	Spores − Mycobacteria + Bacteria + Viruses+	Noncritical equipment, floors, walls, furnishings	Not required	Safe for environment, nontoxic, rapid action, active in the presence of organic materials, excellent cleaning ability due to detergent properties	Contraindicated for use on copper, brass, carbon-tipped devices, and anodized aluminum
4	Iodophors	Disruption of protein and nucleic acid structure and synthesis	Spores − Mycobacteria + Bacteria + Viruses+	Hydrotherapy tanks, thermometers, hard surfaces and equipment that do not touch mucous membranes (IV poles, wheelchairs, beds, call bells)	Not required	Nontoxic, rapid action	Corrosive to metal unless combined with inhibitors; inactivated by organic materials; may stain fabrics and synthetic materials

(continued)

Table 10.3 (continued)

S. no.	Disinfectant	Mode of action	Microbicidal activity	Uses	Monitoring	Advantages/comments	Disadvantages/comments
5	Phenolics	Act as protoplasmic poison, i.e., penetrate and disrupt the cell wall and precipitate the cell proteins, inactivation of essential enzyme systems, and leakage of essential metabolites from the cell wall	Spores – Mycobacteria+ Bacteria+ Viruses+	Disinfection of environmental surfaces (floors, walls, furnishings) and noncritical medical devices (IV poles, wheelchairs, beds, call bells)	Not required	Leaves residual film on environmental surfaces, commercially available with added detergents to provide one-step cleaning and disinfecting	Do not use in nurseries due to risk of hyperbilirubinemia; toxic if inhaled; corrosive
6	Quaternary ammonium compounds (QUATs)	Inactivation of energy-producing enzymes, denaturation of essential cell proteins, and disruption of the cell membrane	Spores – Mycobacteria – Bacteria+ Viruses+	Floors, walls, and furnishings; blood pressure cuffs	Not required	Noncorrosive, nontoxic, low irritant, good cleaning ability, usually have detergent properties, rinsing not required	Not to be used to disinfect instruments; narrow microbicidal spectrum; may be neutralized by various materials (e.g., gauze)

– (not effective), + (effective)

organizations such as the American College of Gastroenterology, the Society of Gastroenterology Nurses and Associates, and the Association for Professionals in Infection Control and Epidemiology. The published recommendations for cleaning and disinfection of endoscopes need to be strictly followed in letter and spirit. To ensure that reprocessing personnel are properly trained, each person who reprocesses endoscopic instruments should receive initial and annual competency testing. In general, after dissembling a scope, the following steps are to be followed to ensure the scopes are free of microbial contamination to control nosocomial infections:

I. *Pre-cleaning*: It removes patient biomaterial and microorganisms from the endoscope. To avoid additional delays, the endoscope insertion tube should be wiped down and all of the channels flushed with detergent and/or water (as specified by manufacturer's instructions) as soon after the procedure as possible, preferably immediately. The mechanical action of wiping the endoscope with appropriate detergent solution, coupled with flushing all of the channels, removes biomaterial that harbors and provides nutrients for microorganisms. If pre-cleaning is not initiated within an hour, the endoscope should be soaked in an appropriate enzymatic detergent according to the manufacturer's recommendations, before mechanical cleaning and then terminal reprocessing. This process will allow for any dried debris to be loosened and ensure its removal during cleaning.

II. *Mechanical cleaning*: After point-of-use pre-cleaning, transport the soiled endoscope to the reprocessing area before the remaining soil dries. Perform pressure/leak testing before formal reprocessing. Meticulous cleaning of the entire endoscope, including valves, channels, connectors, and all detachable parts, must precede any sterilization or high-level disinfection procedure. Failure to perform good cleaning can result in sterilization or disinfection failure, and outbreaks of infection can occur. Disassemble the parts as far as possible, and completely immerse the scope and components in an appropriate detergent that is compatible with the endoscope, according to the manufacturer's instructions. Use of the specific dilution of the detergents and submerging the endoscope completely for the required length of time are essential to ensure the efficacy of the procedure. Use of enzymatic detergent is recommended to help break down and flush patient biomaterial from the scope. Cleaning reduces the level of microbial contamination by 4–6 $\log_{10}$ [13]. The recommended sink/basin should be at least 16 in. by 16 in. by 8 in.. Use brushes appropriate for the size of the endoscope channel, parts, connectors, and orifices (e.g., bristles should contact all surfaces) for cleaning. Items used for cleaning should be disposable or thoroughly cleaned and disinfected/sterilized between uses.

III. *Disinfection/sterilization:* High-level disinfection or sterilization of endoscopes is listed as a requirement in all guidelines. Ethylene oxide sterilization of flexible endoscopes is infrequent because it requires a lengthy processing and aeration time (e.g., 12 h) and a potential hazard to staff and patients. High-level disinfection/sterilization with liquid chemicals cleared by FDA is the standard. At this time, the FDA-cleared formulations include $\geq$2.4 % glutaraldehyde, 0.55 % orthophthalaldehyde (OPA), 0.95 % glutaraldehyde with 1.64 % phenol/phenate, 7.35 % hydrogen peroxide with 0.23 % peracetic acid, 1.0 % hydrogen peroxide with 0.08 % peracetic acid, and 7.5 % hydrogen peroxide. Disinfectants that are not FDA cleared should not be used for reprocessing endoscopes which include iodophors, chlorine solutions, alcohols, quaternary ammonium compounds, and phenolics because of lack of proven efficacy against all microorganisms or materials incompatibility [5]. After high-level disinfection, rinse the endoscope and flush the channels with sterile, filtered, or tap water to remove the disinfectant solution. Discard the rinse water after each use/cycle. Flush the channels with 70–90 % ethyl or isopropyl alcohol and dry by using forced air.

Automated endoscope reprocessor (AER) available offers several advantages over manual reprocessing: they automate and standardize several important reprocessing steps, reduce the likelihood that an essential reprocessing step will be skipped, and reduce personnel exposure to high-level disinfectants or chemical sterilants. At the same time, failure of AER has been linked to outbreaks of infections or colonization. Establishment of correct connectors between the AER and the device is critical to ensure complete flow of disinfectant and rinse water.

IV. *Storage*: Store the endoscopes in a way that prevents recontamination and promotes drying (e.g., hung vertically). Endoscopes should be stored in a clean, dry, and well-ventilated area to minimize the possibility of recontamination. Also, all valves and the water-resistant cap should be removed during storage to facilitate drying. Although reuse of endoscopes within 10–14 days of high-level disinfection appears to be safe, the data are insufficient to provide a maximal duration for use of appropriately cleaned, reprocessed, dried, and stored flexible endoscopes. This interval remains poorly defined and warrants further study.

Monitoring of Disinfection Process

The process of high-level disinfection requires monitoring and auditing [14]:
1. Commercially available chemical test strips should be used to determine whether an effective concentration of active ingredients of disinfectant is present, despite repeated use and dilution.
   - The frequency of testing should be based on frequency of use of the solutions (i.e., test daily if used daily).
   - Chemical test strips must be verified for their accuracy each time a new package/bottle is opened, using appropriate positive (e.g., full strength disinfectant solution) and negative (e.g., tap water) controls, as

per manufacturer's recommendations for disinfectants.
   - A disinfectant solution should not be used beyond the expiration date, irrespective of results of test strips.
   - Prepared solutions shall not be topped up with fresh solution.
   - If manual disinfection is performed, the container used for disinfection shall be kept covered during use and washed, rinsed, and dried when the solution is changed.
2. A permanent record of processing shall be completed and retained according to the policy of the facility; this record shall include, but not be limited to:
   - The identification of the equipment/device to be disinfected.
   - Date and time of the clinical procedure.
   - Concentration and contact time of the disinfectant used in each process.
   - Results of each inspection (and, for endoscopes, each leak test).
   - Result of each testing of the disinfectant and the name of the person completing the reprocessing.
   - Disinfection practices shall be audited on a regular basis and a quality improvement process must be in place to deal with any irregularities/concerns resulting from the audit.

Sterilization

There are a variety of sterilizing methods suitable for healthcare facilities including steam sterilization (autoclaving), dry heat sterilization, and low-temperature sterilizing processes (ethylene oxide, peracetic acid, and hydrogen peroxide plasma). The sterilization method chosen must be compatible with the item to be sterilized to avoid damage. Manufacturer's recommendations are to be followed when determining the method of sterilization for individual items.

(A) *Steam Sterilization*

The basic principle of steam sterilization, as accomplished in an autoclave, is to expose each item to direct steam contact at the required temperature and pressure for the specified time.

Steam sterilization is nontoxic, inexpensive, rapidly microbicidal, and sporicidal and rapidly heats and penetrates fabrics. Moist heat destroys microorganisms by the irreversible coagulation and denaturation of enzymes and structural proteins by the principle of condensation; thereby process of condensation acts as the sterilant in steam sterilization. In healthcare facilities, four generic types of steam sterilizers may be found:

- Downward displacement steam sterilizer: Steam is admitted at the top or the sides of the sterilizing chamber and, because the steam is lighter than air, forces air out from the bottom of the chamber through the vent drain. The gravity displacement autoclaves are primarily used to process laboratory media, water, pharmaceutical products, regulated medical waste, and nonporous articles whose surfaces have direct steam contact.
- Prevacuum steam sterilizer (for porous and cannulated loads) is similar to the gravity displacement sterilizers except they are fitted with a vacuum pump (or ejector) to ensure air removal from the sterilizing chamber and load before the steam is admitted. An air-removal test (Bowie-Dick test) must be performed daily in an empty dynamic air-removal sterilizer (e.g., prevacuum steam sterilizer) to ensure air removal. A commercially available Bowie-Dick-type test sheet should be placed in the center of the *challenge pack* in an otherwise empty chamber and run at 134 °C for 3.5 min. The test is used each day the vacuum-type steam sterilizer is used, before the first processed load. Sterilizer vacuum performance is acceptable if the sheet inside the test pack shows a uniform color change. Entrapped air will cause a spot to appear on the test sheet, due to the inability of the steam to reach the chemical indicator. If the sterilizer fails the Bowie-Dick test, take the sterilizer out of service till it is examined by the sterilizer maintenance personnel and passes a repeat Bowie-Dick-type test [15, 16]. The Bowie-Dick is not applicable to downward displacement sterilizers as these have a longer cycle which can cause change to the indicator even when there is air present.

- Steam-flush pressure-pulsing process, which removes air rapidly by repeatedly alternating a steam flush and a pressure pulse above atmospheric pressure. Air is rapidly removed from the load as with the prevacuum sterilizer, but air leaks do not affect this process because the steam in the sterilizing chamber is always above atmospheric pressure.
- Benchtop steam sterilizer (which is only suitable for porous loads if it has a suitable drying stage).

Steam quality [8]: Steam quality affects the degree of sterilization and dryness of processed materials. There are three categories of steam quality that will hinder the efficacy of the sterilization process:

- Moisture content of steam (dryness fraction): Steam should be not too wet and not too dry. Excess moisture carried in the steam may cause wet loads, while superheated steam is a problem for reliable sterilization because it is dry and needs to cool before its moisture (necessary for fast killing of microorganisms) becomes available. The moisture content of the steam (dryness fraction) is measured as the weight of dry steam present in a mixture of dry saturated steam and contained water. Ideal steam for sterilization is 100 % dry saturated steam, although in practice, values greater than 97 % are considered acceptable. Steam in the sterilizer may become superheated during expansion into the chamber from a much higher pressure, or it may be produced through malfunction of sterilizer or steam supply components.
- Noncondensable gases, e.g., air content of steam: Noncondensable gases are those which do not exhibit a change between gas and liquid states in the normal operating range of temperatures of a steam sterilizer. They seriously interfere with the heat plus moisture conditions necessary for microbial death. Air is generally "incondensable" and may be trapped in steam being delivered to a sterilizer. Other noncondensable gases may arise from boiler water treatment regimens or residues of chemicals used to treat the interior of steam supply pipes. Noncondensable gas entrainment can be minimized though the correct chemical

treatment of boiler water. The removal of noncondensable gases can be facilitated by the installation of air vent assemblies at high points on the steam line before the sterilizer.

- Particulate or chemical contamination carried in the steam arising from an impure water supply (from which the steam is generated) or improper operation of the boiler or steam generator.

Steam quality testing: Steam quality testing is recommended during the commissioning of a sterilizer and or steam boiler to establish baseline data. The *load dryness test* may be carried out by comparing the dryness of a load of sterilized porous articles, after they have returned to ambient temperature following the sterilization process, with the dryness of similar porous articles which have not been sterilized, at the same temperature.

Flash sterilization: Flash sterilization is a modification of conventional steam sterilization (either gravity, prevacuum, or steam-flush pressure-pulse) in which the flashed item is placed in an open tray or is placed in a specially designed, covered, rigid container to allow for rapid penetration of steam. The Association for the Advancement of Medical Instrumentation (AAMI) defines flash sterilization as the process designed for the steam sterilization of patient care items for immediate use [17]. This is not recommended as a routine sterilization method because of the lack of rapid-read biological indicators to monitor performance, absence of protective packaging following sterilization, possibility for contamination of processed items during transportation to operating rooms, and the use of minimum sterilization parameters. For this many hospitals have installed the equipment for flash sterilization in close proximity to operating rooms, and new biological indicators that provide results in 1–3 h are available for flash sterilized items.

"Flash" Sterilization Recommendations

- Restrict use to emergencies, such as unexpected surgery or dropped instruments.

- "Flash" sterilizers must never be used for in-house implantables, suction tubing or cannulas, or any other product not specifically validated for the "flash" process. Commercially available presterilized implants, however, are re-sterilized rapidly using this method.

(B) *Dry Heat Sterilization*

Dry heat is less effective than moist heat. This method should be used only for materials that might be damaged by moist heat or that are impenetrable to moist heat (e.g., powders, petroleum products, sharp instruments). The hot air oven working at 160–180 $^\circ$ C with a holding time of 30–120 min can be used for mixed loads of glass and metal instruments and also for some sharp instruments in ophthalmic surgery.

Advantages of dry heat sterilization include [8] the following:
- Nontoxic
- Environment friendly
- For sterilizing goods which are impossible to dry in a steam sterilizer or which may be damaged/corroded by the moisture of steam sterilization
- Low operating costs

Disadvantages of dry heat sterilization are as follows:
- Long time involved in heating, sterilizing, and cooling goods
- Possible damage to packaging materials or to some of the items themselves arising from the high temperatures
- Greatest potential for injury to personnel following contact with parts of the sterilizer or the goods being processed

Monitoring of Dry Heat Sterilization

- Temperature measurement needs to be done using thermocouples.
- Biological indicators: *B. atrophaeus* spores to be used to monitor the process.

(C) *Low-Temperature Sterilization Processes*

There are three low-temperature sterilization processes identified for use in healthcare facilities to sterilize items at temperatures of 55 °C or lower. The active sterilants of these processes are ethylene oxide, hydrogen peroxide plasma, and peracetic acid. The immediate advantage of the low-temperature processes is that heat-sensitive items can be sterilized within healthcare facilities.

1. *Ethylene Oxide (ETO)*

ETO is a colorless gas that is inflammable, highly toxic, and explosive. It is used to sterilize heat- or moisture-sensitive medical equipment. The microbicidal activity of ETO is considered to be the result of alkylation of protein, DNA, and RNA. Alkylation, or the replacement of a hydrogen atom with an alkyl group, within cells prevents normal cellular metabolism and replication. The main disadvantages associated with ETO are the lengthy cycle time, the cost, and its potential hazards to patients and staff. Occupation and Health Safety Administration (OSHA) has established a permissible exposure limit (PEL) of 1 ppm airborne ETO in the workplace, expressed as a time-weighted average (TWA) for an 8-h work shift in a 40-h workweek. The "action level" for ETO is 0.5 ppm, expressed as an 8-h TWA, and the short-term excursion limit is 5 ppm, expressed as a 15-min TWA [18]. The four essential parameters (operational ranges) for ETO sterilizers are as follows:

- Gas concentration (450–1,200 mg/l)
- Temperature (37–63 °C)
- Relative humidity (40–80 %) (water molecules carry ETO to reactive sites)
- Exposure time (1–6 h)

The basic ETO sterilization cycle consists of five stages (i.e., preconditioning and humidification, gas introduction, exposure, evacuation, and air washes) and it takes approximately 2 1/2 h excluding aeration time. Mechanical aeration for 8–12 h at 50–60 °C allows desorption of the toxic ETO residue contained in exposed absorbent materials.

2. *Hydrogen Peroxide Gas Plasma*

This is a new sterilization technology, marketed first in 1993 in the United States. "Plasma" is matter excited to a higher energy state than its gaseous form. After air removal from the sterilization chamber by a very deep vacuuming and introduction of hydrogen peroxide solution from a cassette, sterilization is achieved through generation of a plasma of hydrogen peroxide vapor (concentration 6 mg/l) within the load by radio-frequency excitation. The proposed mechanism of action of this device is the production of free radicals within a plasma field that are capable of interacting with essential cell components (e.g., enzymes, nucleic acids). At the end of the cycle, hydrogen peroxide vapor is replaced by filtered air, and the hydrogen peroxide vapor is converted back into water and oxygen. Automated machines using hydrogen peroxide plasma to chemically process medical and surgical instruments are currently available. The total processing time varies from 52 to 73 min depending upon the type of sterilizer being used. This method is normally used for wrapped items and endoscopes.

3. *Peracetic acid*: Peracetic acid is a highly biocidal oxidizer which denatures proteins, disrupts cell wall permeability, and oxidizes sulfhydryl and sulfur bonds in proteins, enzymes, and other metabolites. An automated machine using peracetic acid is used to chemically sterilize medical (e.g., GI endoscopes) and surgical (e.g., flexible endoscopes) instruments in the United States. The sterilant, 35 % peracetic acid, and an anticorrosive agent are supplied in a single-dose container. The concentrated peracetic acid is diluted to 0.2 % with filtered water (0.2 μm) at a temperature of approximately 50 °C. The diluted peracetic acid is circulated within the chamber of the machine and pumped through the channels of the endoscope for 12 min, decontaminating exterior surfaces, lumens, and accessories [19]. The peracetic acid is discarded via the sewer and the instrument rinsed four times with filtered water. Clean filtered air is passed through the chamber of the machine and endoscope channels to remove excess water. The use of biological monitors (*G. stearothermophilus* spore strips) is recommended by the manufacturers to ensure effectiveness of the process.

4. *Ionizing radiation*: These methods are not available for use in hospitals, but are commonly used commercially (e.g., for disposable syringes).

Monitoring of Sterilization

Monitoring is required when a sterilizer is first installed before it is put into general use and while on routine use:

1. *Physical monitors*: A physical monitor is a device that monitors the physical parameters of a sterilizer, such as time, temperature, and pressure, which are measured during the sterilization cycle and recorded (as a printout or electronic record) on the completion of each cycle.

2. *Biological indicators (BI)*: A biological indicator is a test system containing viable microorganisms (e.g., spore-laden strips or vials) providing a defined resistance to a specified sterilization process. Once sterilized, a BI is incubated to see if the microorganism will grow, which indicates a failure of the sterilizer. **Load Control** is a process by which a load is monitored and released on the basis of a biological indicator in a test pack. *B. atrophaeus* (formerly *Bacillus subtilis*) spores (10^6) are used to monitor ETO and dry heat, and *G. stearothermophilus* spores (10^5) are used to monitor steam sterilization, hydrogen peroxide gas plasma, and liquid peracetic acid sterilizers. *G. stearothermophilus* is incubated at 55–60 °C, and *B. atrophaeus* is incubated at 35–37 °C.

Challenge pack [5]: The size and composition of the biological indicator test pack should be standardized to create a significant challenge to air removal and sterilant penetration and to obtain interpretable results:

- *Steam sterilizers*: 16 freshly laundered reusable absorbent surgical towels each of which is approximately 40 cm by 65 cm are used. Each towel is folded along its length into thirds and widthwise in the middle. The folded towels are placed one top on the other to form a stack 15 cm in height and it should weigh approximately 1.5 kg. The biological indicator is placed between the seventh and eighth towels in the center of the pack. The pack is then taped with two rounds of tape. Place the pack at cold point, which is normally in the front and bottom near the drain.

- *ETO sterilization*: The test pack should be made up by placing one biological indicator in a plastic syringe of sufficient size so that the plunger diaphragm does not touch the indicator when the plunger is inserted into the barrel. The needle end of the syringe must be opened. These items are then placed in a wrapper or a peel pouch which is large enough to contain the test pack components. Prior to assembly the test pack components should be held at 18–24 °C at 35 % relative humidity for at least 2 h.

The BI is incubated according to the manufacturer's instructions. Most BIs require up to 48 h of incubation before the test is complete. Recently, however, *rapid readout biological indicators* have become available that provide BI results in 1 h.

3. *Chemical Indicators (CI)* [20]: A chemical indicator is a system that responds to a change in one or more predefined process variables with a chemical or physical change. Chemical indicators do not necessarily indicate that a device is sterile and do not replace the need to use a BI, but do indicate that the package has been processed through a sterilization cycle. As per the Association for the Advancement of Medical Instrumentation [20], there are six classes of chemical indicators:

Class I: Process indicators differentiate processed from non-processed items. These are applied externally on individual packs and respond to one or more critical process variables, e.g., indicator tapes, labels, and load cards.

Class II: Indicator for use in specific test procedures as defined in sterilizer/sterilization standards (e.g., air detection, steam penetration). These are used for equipment control to evaluate the sterilizer performance, e.g., Bowie-Dick test.

Class III: Single-variable indicator that reacts to a single critical variable in the sterilization process to indicate when a stated value has been reached (e.g., temperature at a specific location in the chamber). These are used for pack control and exposure control monitoring, e.g., temperature tubes.

Class IV: Multivariable indicator that reacts to two or more critical variables in the sterilization cycle is used for pack control, e.g., paper strips.

Class V: Integrating indicator that reacts to all critical variables in the sterilization cycle (time, temperature, presence of steam) and has stated values that correlate to a BI at three time/temperature relationships. This responds to critical variables in the same way that a BI responds and is equivalent to the performance requirements of BIs. It is used for pack control and can be used as an additional tool to release loads that do not contain implants.

Class VI: Emulating indicator that reacts to all critical variables for a specified sterilization cycle (e.g., 10, 18, 40 min); a different one is needed for each cycle. This is used as internal CI for pack control but cannot be used as an additional tool to release loads that do not contain implants.

Process challenge device (PCD) [5]: A process challenge device simulates the worst-case conditions for the attainment of the specified sterilizing conditions within items to be sterilized. The device is so constructed that a biological or chemical indicator can be placed within the device in the position, which is the most difficult for the sterilizing agent to reach. Monitoring of sterilization of small lumen devices is done using PCDs. The design of the process challenge device depends on the nature of goods to be sterilized and the sterilization procedure. During routine monitoring of sterilizers, the BI and/or CI is usually placed within a PCD and placed in the sterilizer. A PCD can be commercially manufactured or prepared in-house.

Indicator shall be used only for the sterilizer type and cycle for which it was designed and validated and stored according to the indicator manufacturer's instructions and shall not be used beyond the expiration date.

Routine Monitoring

- Document daily operation of the sterilizer: Review physical monitoring parameters for each operation (e.g., printed or electronic

records). The mechanical monitors for steam sterilizers and ETO include temperature and cycle time and temperature and pressure, respectively. Generally, two essential elements for ETO sterilization (i.e., the gas concentration and humidity) cannot be monitored in healthcare ETO sterilizers.

- Each package to be sterilized shall have an externally visible chemical indicator (*Exposure Control*), which is examined immediately after sterilization to make sure that the item has been exposed to the sterilization process.
- Preferably, a chemical indicator also should be placed on the inside of each pack to verify sterilant penetration (*Inside Pack Control*).
- Steam and low-temperature sterilizers (e.g., hydrogen peroxide gas plasma, peracetic acid) should be monitored at least weekly with the appropriate biological indicator.
- A biological indicator shall be included in every load containing implantable devices
- A biological indicator shall be included in every load that is to be sterilized with ethylene oxide.
- Biological indicators specifically designed for monitoring flash sterilization are now available and should be only used as others do not provide reliable monitoring of flash sterilizers.
- Retain sterilization records (mechanical, chemical, and biological) for a minimum period as recommended by regulatory authorities.

Failure of a BI

Since sterilization failure can occur (about 1 % for steam), a procedure to follow in the event of positive spore tests with steam sterilization has been suggested by CDC [5] (Fig. 10.1). For sterilization methods other than steam (e.g., ETO, hydrogen peroxide gas plasma), a more conservative approach has been recommended in which even a single positive spore test (excepting a defective BI) is assumed to represent sterilizer malfunction and requires that all materials processed in that sterilizer must be considered non-sterile and retrieved, if possible, and reprocessed.

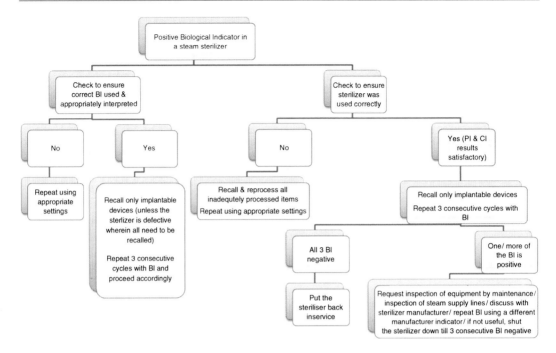

Fig. 10.1 Suggested protocol for management of positive BI in a steam sterilizer

Parametric Release

In Europe, BI is not used routinely to monitor the sterilization process. Instead, release of sterilizer items is based on monitoring the physical conditions of the sterilization process that is termed "parametric release." Parametric release requires that there is a defined quality system in place at the facility performing the sterilization and that the sterilization process be validated for the items being sterilized. At present in Europe, parametric release is accepted for steam, dry heat, and ionizing radiation processes, as the physical conditions are understood and can be monitored directly [21].

Traceability and recall process: A healthcare facility needs clear policies and procedures in place to minimize the likelihood that medical devices improperly processed within the facility are released for patient use and to ensure that suspected non-sterile medical devices that have been released are recalled in a timely manner. There should be an established "recall" procedure in each facility, the objective of which is to "expedite the retrieval of processed items that are

suspected to be non-sterile and to ensure adequate follow-up actions such as quarantine of the sterilizer, notification of physicians and affected clinical departments, and surveillance of patients." [15] Recall policies and procedures should address documentation and records maintenance. The recall procedures should:

- Be written
- Outline the circumstances for issuing a recall order
- Designate the person(s) authorized to issue a recall order
- Designate the person(s) responsible for reporting on the execution of a recall order

Shelf Life and Event-Related Sterility

It is impossible to recommend a universal standard for the duration a sterile package can remain sterile due to enormous variations from hospital to hospital [5]. This means that in charge of this activity must establish and justify their practices.

For years, the subject of expiration dating has generated considerable debate. Many hospitals have considered 30 days to be the standard time period for dating hospital wrapped sterile supplies, principally because of 1971 and 1973 shelf-life studies conducted by the CDC. Those results indicated that items double-wrapped in muslin had a shelf life of 3 weeks and that packs stored in dust covers were considered sterile for at least 9 months. New and improved packaging materials, along with greater understanding of the factors affecting sterility, have fueled the debate over expiration dating. Changes in accreditation standards reflect the premise that contamination is "event related" and not "time related" and recognize the hospital's expertise in maintaining and delivering sterile products. The following professional organizations recommend practices that do not require time-related expiration dating:

- Association for the Advancement of Medical Instrumentation, Joint Commission on Accreditation of Healthcare Organisations, Association of Operating Room Nurses, USA (AAMI, JCAHO,AORN, 1993)

Event-related sterility Policy defines procedures intended to maintain the sterility of packages until they are used. This relates to the sterility of hospital-prepared packages containing sterile supplies wrapped in single-use or reusable materials. Since some supplies have expiration dates and degrade over time, this covers only those supplies for which the manufacturer or the distributor does not provide expiration dating in the form of labeling, instructions of use, or other statements.

Shelf life: The shelf life of a packaged sterile item is event-related and depends on the following:

1. The quality of the wrapper material
2. The storage conditions
3. The conditions during transport
4. The amount of handling (punctured packaging, dropping on floor, rough handling, bending, creasing, getting wet or damp, etc.)

Ideally, sterile storage areas should be air-conditioned with minimal air turbulence created by fans. The following points are minimum requirements whether or not storage conditions are air-conditioned:

- Area to be dedicated for sterile stock storage
- Free from dust, insects, and vermin
- Temperature range to be between 18 °C and 22 °C with a relative humidity ranging from 35 % to 68 %

With the change in accreditation standards, hospitals are now able to develop procedures that more accurately reflect their sterile containment needs. Clear direction that final inspection of the package and the ultimate decision to use the contents rests with the user. There should be written policies and procedures for how shelf life is determined and for how it is indicated on the product, e.g.:

- Expiration dating: "Each item intended for use as a sterile product must be labeled with a lot control number, date of sterilization and for stock rotation, and the following statement: 'Product is not sterile if packaging is open, damaged, or wet. Please check before using.'"

Time-related sterilization can also be added to the event-related sterility. In most hospitals 6 months are given under ideal storing conditions beyond which the item is reprocessed or discarded.

Reuse of Single-Use Medical Devices

The reprocessing and reuse of single-use medical devices is a common practice, although many scientific bodies and establishments advise against this [22]. It is often justified on the basis of economic and environmental benefits. However, these perceived benefits are questionable as many of the processes required to ensure that the device is safe and fit for its intended use cannot be undertaken by the reprocessor (a person who undertakes the reprocessing of a medical device). Many single-use devices are reused without adequate evaluation of the increased risks to patients. We want to draw attention to the pitfalls and risks associated with reprocessing and reusing single-use medical devices. The issue of reuse of single-use devices is often discussed in resource-poor countries. Research over such issues is very limited. Having said that, this is also equally true that it may be lifesaving for a patient not able to afford an off-the-shelf balloon for angioplasty but can afford a reusable device which may cost only a fraction of its original and save lives. There is paucity of data on a randomized control trial in this direction because such studies may not be viewed favorably by the ethics committee.

The practice of reprocessing single-use devices (SUDs) for reuse began in hospitals in as early as the 1970s. Approval of the practice of reusing hemodialyzers in the early 1980s by the US Public Health Service led the way for current activity.

In the past, single-use devices considered for reprocessing included "outdated" items, based on an arbitrary date-related indicator of sterility. With the current practice of using an event-related sterility indicator (e.g., package damaged or not intact), there are only two categories of single-use items that require consideration for reprocessing.

Historically, most items in the hospitals were designated as reusable and were reprocessed and reused. The use of disposables became popular because of convenience and reducing the risk of cross contamination. However, as the cost of waste disposal increased, hospitals looked for opportunities to reuse waste.

The FDA policy on instrument reuse from 1987 states that the reuse decision belongs to the hospital and the practitioner. In a 1998 letter, the FDA commented on the absence of evidence of adverse patient outcomes related to the reuse of single-use devices. A 1998 survey of OR managers indicated that over a 4-year period, the reuse of single-use devices almost doubled. The increase in reuse of single-use items raised questions about patient safety, informed consent, and the need for equitable regulation of the original equipment manufacturer and the reprocessors. In February 2000, the FDA released the draft document "Reprocessing and Reuse of Single-Use Devices: Review Prioritization Scheme" and in August 14, 2000, released a guidance document, "Enforcement Priorities for Single-Use Devices Reprocessed by Third Parties and Hospitals." These publications followed a period of intense discussion between the FDA and stakeholders and created opportunities for all parties to provide information to the FDA.

In the August 14, 2000, guidance document, the FDA reexamined its policy on the issue of reuse of medical devices labeled for single use with the primary goal of protecting the health of the public by assuring that the practice of reprocessing and reusing single-use devices (SUDs) is safe and effective and based on good science. Subsequent documents have been published by the FDA in 2003 and 2005 to provide guidance for the industry and FDA staff to supplement and clarify related guidance and regulations and are available at the FDA Reuse Web site. Since these 2,000 guidance documents were issued, hospitals have transferred their in-house reprocessing to third-party reprocessors, and in an FDA survey conducted in February 2002, it was found that 24 % of hospitals were using at least one type of reprocessed SUD and the majority of them used "third parties" to reprocess their SUDs.

Key points remain

- A device designated as "single-use" must not be reused but discarded after single procedure. It is not intended to be reprocessed and used again, even on the same patient.
- The reuse of single-use devices can affect their safety, performance, and effectiveness, exposing patients and staff to unnecessary risk.

Once a device is reused the responsibility for its safety and effectiveness shifts to the institution that undertakes its reuse. It is not possible to restore the device to its original position, but the question arises as to how we handle this compelling desire to reuse a single-use device.

The authors have tried to make a case to the reader where scope for review will always remain. The checks and balances recommended cannot be unlimited whereby the cost-benefit ratio is lost. The concerns that arise out of such activity are as below:

1. Ethical.
2. Maintenance of the quality of the product to an acceptable limit.
3. Can the device sustain the process which may render it reusable?
4. Can the product be rendered sterile for human use?

5. Consent from the patient or the relatives in unconscious patients.
6. Number of times a specific device can be reused. Factors that impact cycle turns are the reprocessing method, durability of the manufacturer's device, and the staff handling the device.

Most problems caused by reuse of a single-use device may fall into one or more of the following areas.

1. *Potential for Cross Infection*

   Due to design, e.g., narrow lumens and the type of material used, e.g., heat-sensitive materials, viable microorganisms may be incompletely removed and be transferred to the next patient.

2. *Inability to Clean and Decontaminate*

   It is well known that any disinfection or sterilization to be effective the device needs to be prior cleaned adequately. This process should be validated, to establish that it will consistently provide results complying with its predetermined specifications. Examples of features of a device that make cleaning difficult are acute angles, coils, long or narrow lumens, specialist surface coatings, etc.

3. *Residues from Chemical Decontamination Agents*

   Some materials used in device manufacture can absorb or adsorb certain chemicals, which can then gradually leach from the material over time, resulting in chemical burns or a risk of sensitization of the patient or the user.

4. *Material Alteration*

   Exposure to chemical agents, such as cleaning agents and chemical sterilants, may cause corrosion and/or changes in the materials of the device. Exposure to elevated temperatures or pressure during the sterilization process may also alter the properties or cause degradation of the device material. For example, plastics may soften, crack, or become brittle.

5. *Mechanical Failure*

   Some devices may experience stress during each cycle of reuse, leading to fatigue-induced failure and fracturing, e.g., single-use drill burrs, saw blades, and craniotomy blades.

6. *Reactions to Endotoxins*

   Endotoxins from Gram-negative bacterial breakdown products can be an issue if the device has a heavy bacterial load after use, which cannot be adequately removed by cleaning. The sterilization process will not inactivate the toxins, even when cleaning and sterilization is effective in killing the bacteria. Moreover, monitoring of sterilization for small lumen devices also is a specialized area.

7. *Prion Diseases*

   Prions, the abnormal proteins associated with prion diseases (e.g., Creutzfeldt-Jakob disease (CJD) and variant Creutzfeldt-Jakob disease (vCJD)) are very resistant to all conventional methods of decontamination. In order to reduce the risk of transmission of abnormal prion proteins during surgical procedures, the Department of Health issued advice describing the present state of knowledge of the risks of transmission of vCJD from one patient to another. Health Service Circular 1999/178, vCJD: Minimising the Risk of Transmission [23], states that "devices designated for single episodes of use must not be reused under any circumstances whatsoever." In addition, the Advisory Committee on Dangerous Pathogens (ACDP) TSE Risk Management Subgroup published guidelines in 2003 – "Transmissible Spongi-form Encephalopathy Agents: Safe Working and the Prevention of Infection." [24] It has been updated and many annexes added since 2003 as more scientific information has become available.

Conclusions

To conclude, the decontamination and sterilization procedures in any healthcare setting is a serious business that needs checks, and balances throughout the process in the procedures are defined and monitored regularly. The safety of patients in any healthcare settings can get compromised, once the policy and SOP are generated in decontamination and sterilization procedures. One of the important entities ensuring welfare of the patients admitted to a hospital are taken care of to a large extent and NABH accreditation of the hospital gets considerably easy. Authors have tried to present to the readers the various internationally accepted procedures and guidelines that needs to be followed. The concept of event-related sterility and reuse of device is a thought-provoking topic and has been handled with all sensitivity of a developing world. Quality care can be delivered if the abovementioned procedures and guidelines are followed in letter and spirit.

References

1. Cullen KA, Hall MJ, Golosinskiy A. Ambulatory Surgery in the United States, 2006. National health statistics reports; no 11. Revised. Hyattsville: National Center for Health Statistics. 2009. http://www.cdc.gov/nchs/data/nhsr/nhsr011.pdf
2. Chadha R, Grover M, Sharma A, Lakshmy A, Deb M, Kumar A, Mehta G. An outbreak of post-surgical wound infections due to *Mycobacterium* abscessus. Pediatr Surg Int. 1998;13(5–6):406–10.
3. Veena Kumari HB, Nagarathna S, Chandramouli BA, Umamaheshwara Rao GS, Chandramuki A. Investigation of an outbreak of device-related postoperative ventriculitis: a lesson learnt. Indian J Pathol Microbiol. 2008;51(2):301–3.
4. Corne P, Godreuil S, Jean-Pierre H, Jonquet O, Campos J, Jumas-Bilak E, et al. Unusual implication of biopsy forceps in outbreaks of *Pseudomonas aeruginosa* infections and pseudo-infections related to bronchoscopy. J Hosp Infect. 2005;61:20–6.
5. Rutala WA, Weber DJ. Healthcare Infection Control Practices Advisory Committee (HICPAC). Guideline for disinfection and sterilization in healthcare facilities. 2008. Availablefrom: http://www.cdc.gov/ncidod/dhqp/pdf/guidelines/Disinfection_Nov_2008.pdf
6. Spaulding EH. Chemical disinfection of medical and surgical materials. In: Lawrence C, Block SS, editors. Disinfection, sterilization, and preservation. Philadelphia: Lea & Febiger; 1968. p. 517–31.
7. Ontario. Ministry of Health and Long-Term Care and the Provincial Infectious Diseases Advisory Committee. Best practices for cleaning, disinfection and sterilization in all health care settings. 2009. Available at: http://www.health.gov.on.ca/english/providers/program/infectious/diseases/ic_cds.html. Accessed 15 Dec 2012.
8. Disinfection and infection control guidelines. Available at http://www.health.qld.gov.au/chrisp/sterilising/large_document.pdf. Accessed 15 Dec 2012.
9. Hutchisson B, LeBlanc C. The truth and consequences of enzymatic detergents. Gastroenterol Nurs. 2005;28:372–6.
10. Muscarella LF. Dear Los Angeles Times, the risk of disease transmission during gastrointestinal endoscopy. Gastroenterol Nurs. 2004;27:271–8.
11. Ramsey AH, Oemig TV, Davis JP, Massey JP, Torok TJ. An outbreak of bronchoscopy-related *Mycobacterium* tuberculosis infections due to lack of bronchoscope leak testing. Chest. 2002;121:976–81.
12. U.S. Food and Drug Administration. Draft guidance for the content of premarket notifications for endoscopes used in gastroenterology and urology. Rockville: National Press Office; 1995.
13. Martiny H, Floss H, Zuhlsdorf B. The importance of cleaning for the overall results of processing endoscopes. J Hosp Infect. 2004;56 Suppl 2:S16–22.
14. The-ASEAN-Guidelines-for-Disinfection-and-Sterilisation-of-Instruments-in-Health-Care-Facilities. Available from http://apsic.info/documents/The-ASEAN-Guidelines-for-Disinfection-and-Sterilisation-of-Instruments-in-Health-Care-Facilities.pdf. Accessed 15 Dec 2012.
15. Association for the Advancement of Medical Instrumentation. Comprehensive guide to steam sterilization and sterility assurance in health care facilities, ANSI/AAMI ST79. 2006.
16. American Society for Healthcare Central Service Professionals. Training manual for health care central service technicians. In: Association AH, editor. Chicago: The Jossey-Bass/American Hospital Association Press Series; 2001. p. 1–271.
17. The Association for the Advancement of Medical Instrumentation. Flash sterilization of patient care items for immediate use. Arlington: The Association for the Advancement of Medical Instrumentation; 1996. x-16.
18. Association for the Advancement of Medical Instrumentation. Ethylene oxide sterilization in health care facilities: safety and effectiveness. Arlington: AAMI; 1999.
19. Bradley CR, Babb JR, Ayliffe GA. Evaluation of the steris system 1 peracetic acid endoscope processor. J Hosp Infect. 1995;29:143–51.
20. American National Standard. Sterilization of health care products–chemical indicators–Part 1: general requirement ANSI/AAMI/ISO 11140-1. 2005.
21. Baird RM. Sterility assurance: concepts, methods and problems. In: Russell AD, Hugo WB, Ayliffe GAJ, editors. Principles and practice of disinfection, preservation and sterilization. Oxford, UK: Blackwell Scientific Publications; 1999. p. 787–99.
22. MHRA DB 2006(04) v2.0 December 2011. (http://www.mhra.gov.uk/home/groups/dts-iac/documents/publication/con2025021.pdf). Accessed 22 Dec 2012.
23. Department of Health. Health service circular 1999/178, variant Creutzfeldt-Jakob Disease (vCJD): minimising the risk of transmission. http://www.dh.gov.uk/en/Publicationsandstatistics/Lettersandcirculars/Healthservicecirculars/DH_4004969
24. ACDP TSE Risk Management Subgroup guidelines. Transmissible spongiform encephalopathy agents: safe working and the prevention of infection. 2003. http://www.dh.gov.uk/ab/ACDP/TSEguidance/index.htm

Part IX

Monitoring of High-Risk Areas

Monitoring of High-Risk Areas: Intensive Care Units

11

B.K. Rao

Infections in the intensive care unit (ICU) setting constitute one of the greatest challenges of modern medicine especially with the increasing occurrence of infection caused by multidrug-resistant or extremely drug-resistant pathogens. Although device utilization in the developing countries' ICUs is remarkably similar to that reported from US ICUs, rates of device-associated nosocomial infection are reported to be markedly higher in the ICUs of the developing countries' hospitals [1]. Patients requiring ICU care can have community-acquired infections or hospital-acquired infections or healthcare-associated infections. Hospital-acquired infections (HAIs) are a cause of increased morbidity, mortality, and resource expenditure throughout the hospital setting and particularly in the intensive care unit. The severity of underlying disease, invasive diagnostic and therapeutic procedures that breach normal host defenses, contaminated life-support equipment, and the prevalence of resistant microorganisms are critical factors in the high rate of infection in the ICUs.

Critically ill patients are a special subset of patients with predisposition to HAIs. The most common ICU infections are pneumonia, bloodstream infection, and urinary tract infection. The Extended Prevalence of Infection in Intensive Care (EPIC II) study revealed that 51 % of patients were infected on the study day and 71 % of all patients were receiving antibiotics. The total occurrence of the most frequent types of ICU-acquired infection were respiratory tract infections 63.5 %, abdominal infections 19.6 %, bloodstream infections 15.1 %, and renal or urinary tract infections in 14.3 % [2].

One should monitor infection sites, pathogens, risk factors, and patient location within the facility. Also needed is monitoring of the central line and other invasive devices insertion practices that should include hand hygiene, barrier use, and skin preparation practices.

Correct and timely diagnosis is an essential point in the management of infections in ICU. Diagnosing nosocomial infections in critically ill patients admitted to the ICU is a challenge because signs and symptoms are usually nonspecific for a particular infection. Moreover, there is no consensus about the ideal method to diagnose some of the common infections in the ICU settings (e.g., nosocomial pneumonia in ventilated patients, sepsis, fungal bloodstream infections) or, more generally, to identify the patient who is truly infected. The diagnostic workup of the febrile critically ill patient should be guided by the underlying condition of the patient and the clinical suspicion of a specific infection [3].

To monitor nosocomial infections, microbiological samples must be collected and analyzed. Every ICU requires an incumbent surveillance and training program for control of HAI. Outcome measurements that can be monitored are catheter-related bloodstream infections (CRBSIs),

B.K. Rao, M.D. (✉)
Department of Critical Care and Emergency Medicine, Sir Ganga Ram Hospital, New Delhi, India
e-mail: drbkrao@gmail.com

C. Wattal and N. Khardori (eds.), *Hospital Infection Prevention: Principles & Practices*, DOI 10.1007/978-81-322-1608-7_11, © Springer India 2014

ventilator-associated pneumonias (VAPs), and catheter-associated urinary tract infections (CAUTIs). The rates are presented as rates per 1,000 device days. This uniform format is especially valuable to allow benchmarking and comparisons.

Collection of data should be performed using active, patient-based, and prospective surveillance. The healthcare people involved in the process may be many, but the data must be overseen by infection preventionists.

The specific indicators reflecting infection control must be selected after consideration of their attributable morbidity, cost, preventability, and transmission risks.

Bloodstream Infections

Indwelling intravascular catheters are essential in ICU patients. Primary bloodstream infections (BSIs) are laboratory-confirmed bloodstream infections (LCBIs) that are not secondary to a community-acquired infection or a HAI meeting Center for Disease Control and Prevention (CDC)/National Healthcare Safety Network (NHSN) criteria at another body site.

The terms used to describe intravascular catheter-related infections can be confusing because catheter-related bloodstream infection (CRBSI) and central line-associated bloodstream infection (CLABSI) are often used interchangeably even though the meanings differ. The clinical presentation of a catheter-related infection can be designated as either local (site inflammation, purulent drainage, tenderness) or systemic (bacteremia with or without systemic sepsis). The diagnostic methods used are either simultaneous quantitative blood culture or differential time to positivity blood culture. Assuming that appropriate sterile technique during insertion and appropriate site care has been followed, the presence of entry-site inflammation is neither sensitive nor specific for CRBSI [4].

CRBSI is a clinical definition, used when diagnosing and treating patients, that requires specific laboratory testing that more thoroughly identifies the catheter as the source of the BSI.

It is not typically used for surveillance purposes. CLABSI is a term used by CDC's National Healthcare Safety Network (NHSN) for surveillance purposes and not for clinical management. A CLABSI is a primary BSI in a patient that had a central line within the 48-h period before the development of the BSI and is not bloodstream related to an infection at another site.

Because the purposes of these two definitions differ, the components of the definitions differ. For example, the CRBSI definition includes both the use of catheter-tip cultures and recommends the use of blood cultures drawn through the vascular catheter. The NHSN BSI definition does not utilize catheter-tip cultures nor recommend collecting blood cultures through vascular catheters since not all patients with BSI have catheters.

Several centers monitor adherence to evidence-based central line insertion practices as a method for identifying quality improvement opportunities and strategically targeting interventions.

Ventilator-Associated Pneumonia (VAP)

Ventilator-associated pneumonia (VAP) remains a major challenge in the intensive care unit. Unlike the diagnosis of CABSIs, the case definition for VAP remains controversial. Two broad criteria exist for the diagnosis of VAP. One relies essentially on clinical criteria, while the other requires evidence of a pathogen in the lower airways. Although VAP is being monitored very frequently, wide variation in incidence is possible based on the diagnostic criteria used. Substantial interobserver variability in the clinical criteria for VAP diagnosis is particularly concerning given the way VAP incidence is being utilized as a surrogate for hospital quality. CDC defines ventilator-associated PNEU (VAP) as a pneumonia where the patient is on mechanical ventilation for >2 calendar days when all elements of the PNEU infection criterion were first present together, with day of ventilator placement being Day 1, and the ventilator was in place on the date of event or the day before. If the patient is admitted or transferred into a facility on a ventilator, the day of admission is considered Day 1.The current CDC definition has three specific components: radiologic evidence of infection, systemic findings of inflammation, and specific pulmonary signs of organ compromise. These criteria do not require microbiologic evidence of infection. However, from January 2013 a new protocol for surveillance for ventilator-associated events, including ventilator-associated pneumonia (VAP), in adult patients will be implemented by CDC which will include positive cultures for isolation of the infecting pathogen [5].

New more stringent clinical criteria for VAP have been implemented as part of the National Healthcare Safety Network (NHSN). The new NHSN definition does require isolation of a pathogen. This can derive from blood, pleural, sputum, or lower airway cultures [6].

As none of the currently available diagnostic tests provides an absolute accurate diagnosis of VAP when used alone, a strategy that combines diagnostic modalities is advocated. Patients with suspected VAP should undergo an evaluation that is supported by local expertise and should include imaging procedures (chest radiograph, computed tomography), bacteriologic cultures from the lower respiratory tract, and possibly biomarkers [7].

Since most of the multiresistant organisms (MROs) spread through contact transmission, predominantly by hand transfer, healthcare-associated inpatient MRSA acquisition is a good proxy indicator for compliance of healthcare workers with hand hygiene requirements.

The monitoring of VAP must also include compliance of VAP bundle and antibiotic surveillance.

Catheter-Associated Urinary Tract Infections (CAUTIs)

Urinary catheters often are placed unnecessarily, remain in use without physician awareness, and are not removed promptly when no longer needed. Unlike VAP and CLABSI, catheter-associated urinary tract infections (CAUTIs) increase morbidity more than mortality.

CAUTI is a UTI where an indwelling urinary catheter was in place for >2 calendar days when all elements of the UTI infection criterion were first present together, with day of device placement being Day 1, and an indwelling urinary catheter was in place on the date of event or the day before. Urine cultures must be obtained using appropriate technique, such as clean catch collection or catheterization. Specimens from indwelling catheters should be aspirated through the disinfected sampling ports. Urinary catheter tips should not be cultured and are not acceptable for the diagnosis of a urinary tract infection [8].

CAUTI is a clinical diagnosis characterized by symptoms of infection with positive pus cells and culture positivity. Signs and symptoms compatible with CAUTI include new onset or worsening of fever, rigors, altered mental status, malaise, or lethargy with no other identified cause; flank pain; costovertebral angle tenderness; acute hematuria; pelvic discomfort; and, in those whose catheters have been removed, dysuria, urgent or frequent urination, or suprapubic pain or tenderness. CAUTI in patients with indwelling urethral, indwelling suprapubic, or intermittent catheterization is defined by the presence of symptoms or signs compatible with UTI with no other identified source of infection along with $\geq 10^3$ colony forming units (cfu)/mL of ≥ 1 bacterial species in a single catheter urine specimen or in a midstream voided urine specimen from a patient whose urethral, suprapubic, or condom catheter has been removed within the previous 48 h. Data are insufficient to recommend a specific quantitative count for defining CAUTI in symptomatic men when specimens are collected by condom catheter. In a catheterized patient, pyuria is not diagnostic of CAUTI [9].

References

1. Rosenthal VD, Maki DG, Jamulitrat S, Medeiros EA, Todi SK, Gomez DY, et al. International Nosocomial Infection Control Consortium (INICC) report, data summary for 2003–2008, issued June 2009. Am J Infect Control. 2010;38(2):95–104.
2. Vincent JL, Rello J, Marshall J, Silva E, Anzueto A, Martin CD, Moreno R, Lipman J, Gomersall C, Sakr Y,

Reinhart K. International study of the prevalence and outcomes of infection in intensive care units. JAMA. 2009;302:2323–9.

3. Cruciani M. Meta-analyses of diagnostic tests in infectious diseases: how helpful are they in the intensive care setting? HSR Proc Intensive Care Cardiovasc Anesth. 2011;3:103–8.

4. Safdar N, Maki DG. Inflammation at the insertion site is not predictive of catheter-related bloodstream infection with short-term, noncuffed central venous catheters. Crit Care Med. 2002;30:2632–5.

5. CDC-Ventilator-Associated Event – NHSN. Available at www.cdc.gov/nhsn/psc_da-vae.html

6. Edwards JR, Peterson KD, Mu Y, Banerjee S, Allen-Bridson K, Morrell G, et al. National Healthcare Safety Network (NHSN) report: data summary for 2006 through 2008, issued December 2009. Am J Infect Control. 2009;37:783–805.

7. Morrow LE, Kollef MH. Recognition and prevention of nosocomial pneumonia in the intensive care unit and infection control in mechanical ventilation. Crit Care Med. 2010;38(Suppl):S352–62.

8. Catheter-associated UTI (CAUTI). Available at www.cdc.gov/nhsn/PDFs/pscManual/7psc-CAUTI-current.pdf

9. Hooton TMTM, Bradley SF, Cardenas DD, Colgan R, Geerlings SE, Rice JC, Saint S, Schaeffer AJ, Tambayh PA, Tenke P, Nicolle LE. Diagnosis, prevention, and treatment of catheter-associated urinary tract infection in adults: 2009 international clinical practice guidelines from the Infectious Diseases Society of America. Clin Infect Dis. 2010;50:625–63.

Monitoring of High-Risk Areas: Operating Suite

12

Jayashree Sood and Chand Sahai

Operating suites are very high-risk areas which require regular and high-level monitoring for maintaining high standards of safety. The construction of an operation theater involves meticulous planning such that it prevents airborne microbial contaminants from entering surgical wounds.

Structural changes in the operation theater are not possible once construction is complete. The association between operation theater air quality and postoperative infection is well documented. Therefore, if the ventilation systems that have been installed to supply high-quality air are not satisfactory, there is an increased risk of postoperative infection resulting in unnecessary burden on scarce resources and more importantly patient dissatisfaction. Besides monitoring engineering controls, it is essential to have guidelines for biological controls as well.

Engineering Controls

The master plan should include buffer zones before the entry into the operating rooms [1]. This is where street clothes and shoes are exchanged with the ones earmarked for operating

rooms. Suitable elbow-based sensor scrub stations with a continuous supply of clean water are a must. There should be provision of seamless walls and ceiling with rounded edges in the operation theater. Sliding, instead of swinging, doors should be used so that there is no disturbance of laminar flow. The OT walls and ceiling should be sprayed with antibacterial paint at least 400 µm thick, which does not allow bacteria to grow for a number of years, though this is not a substitute for regular cleaning and carbolization. Maintaining pressure gradient, i.e., high to low, from the operating suite to the corridors with provision of stainless steel cascade stabilizers (Louvers) for continuous monitoring of the pressure gradient is mandatory. A good air-conditioning system (preferably with 100 % fresh air) with at least three filter beds, i.e., pre, micro-V, and HEPA filters (having 99.97 % efficiency), to ensure high quality of air is recommended. Laminar flow is created by providing outlet vents at all four corners of the operating room and periodically tested by the smoke test.

High-efficiency particulate air (HEPA) filters are the terminal filters placed just above the ultraclean zone, which finally filter the incoming air. These filters should be intact, properly seated, and changed at regular intervals and should be able to resist particle penetration from outside (should be able to withhold particles of >3 µm).

J. Sood, M.D., FFARCS, PGDHHM, FICA (✉)
C. Sahai, M.D.
Department of Anaesthesiology, Pain and
Perioperative Medicine, Sir Ganga Ram Hospital,
New Delhi, India
e-mail: jayashreesood@hotmail.com

Monitoring of Engineering Controls

Periodic cleaning of pre and micro-V filters and replacement of HEPA filters should be done after the HEPA filter integrity test has been performed. Monitoring of the incoming air at a proper flow, volume, temperature, and humidity (40–60 %) is essential. At least 20 air changes per hour in the operating suite are mandatory, i.e., the whole volume of the room should be replaced with fresh air, 20 times in 1 h [2]. If the theater has been built with different specifications, the air changes per hour (ACH) should be between 19.5 and 23 [3]. Regular testing of particulate count of the engineering control is essential. It is a better test of filter integrity. Air leaving the final diffuser or filter should contain less than 0.5 (colony forming units) CFU/m^3 of air. An air sample taken close to the wound site should contain less than 10 CFUs/m^3 of air.

The AC ducts should be cleaned periodically using a robotic arm equipment.

Monitoring of Ventilation: The Pressure Differential and Airflow

Monitoring the quality of ventilation is essential with respect to infection control.

Airflow visualization (smoke testing) should be done to ensure appropriate airflow in the operation theater. The test should be done especially around the operating table, wherein the smoke should disperse within seconds. It should be ascertained that the supplied air does not "short circuit," i.e., it should not take a direct route out of the theater wherein it cannot entrain any contamination which is generated in the suite.

Larger airflow patterns can be monitored by using large volume smoke generators. The fire alarm system should be disabled during the smoke testing.

The desired direction of airflow should also be monitored. It should be from the high-pressure operating room to the anesthetic room, disposal room, and lastly the corridor. Pressure differentials between these areas are essential to prevent

backflow of air from the contaminated areas to the operating room. Turbulent airflow with no short-circuiting ensures effective air changes per hour in the operating room. The air exchange rate should be monitored regularly.

The air handling unit, comprising of the humidifier and cooling coil, should be diinfected regularly. To decontaminate the air handling unit, physical cleaning rather than disinfection with microbiological monitoring is recommended.

Air quality monitoring includes annual testing of the ultraclean ventilated theaters. Any malfunction should be reported immediately.

Microbiological Controls and Sampling

An optimal operation room ventilation should prevent airborne microbial contaminants from entering surgical wounds. The main source of these contaminants is the microscopic skin fragments from the operating room staff which get dispersed with movement [4].

Another source is the exposed instruments on which the airborne microorganisms fall [5].

Before being made operational, any operating suite should undergo microbiological sampling (at least 3 samples should be negative before commissioning). Subsequently, the level of airborne bacteria should also be monitored regularly. The ideal time for microbiological testing of an operation theater is just before it comes into use. The air handling unit should be in use at normal flow rates for at least 24 h before sampling. Sampling volumes of approximately 1 m^3 (1,000 L) are optimal. Volumes exceeding 1 m^3 may lead to overcrowding of colonies with difficulty in accurate enumeration and drying of the agar surface due to the increased volume of air passing over it. Sampling volumes less than 1 m^3 may lead to interpretational difficulties and make the data more qualitative. It is important that the bacterial sampler is clean before use. It is recommended that at least three samples per theater should be collected, as this decreases the possibility of technical errors [6].

Microbiological Monitoring

All biomedical waste management principles as per pollution control board guidelines, i.e., segregation of waste at source of generation, treatment at source of generation, safe transportation to the local storage site, proper storage at local site, and ensuring periodic transportation to the final site of disposal, should be observed. Regular training and awareness of staff should be done, regarding infection control practices and procedures to be followed in case of any incident, e.g., needle stick injury. There should be maintenance of proper work, material, and patient flow.

Adequate availability and proper use of personal protective equipment/devices, e.g., cap, mask, gown, and shoe covers, should be confirmed. Ensuring optimum gap time between two surgeries for adequate cleaning of theater should be practiced.

Certain infection control practices which should be observed and practiced in the OT are as follows:

- Spraying of OT table with solution containing alcohol after every surgery.
- Cleaning and carbolization of surfaces with proper cleansing agent and disinfectant, i.e., sodium hypochlorite solution 0.1–1 %.
- Observing surgical hand wash/hand-hygiene guidelines.
- Ensuring proper preparation, use, monitoring, and disposal of high-level disinfectant, e.g., glutaraldehyde or glutaraldehyde OPA solution. The prepared solution should be checked at least once daily for its effectiveness and the availability of free 1.5 % glutraldehyde [7].
- The sterilization process comprises preparation and packing, the actual sterilization process, storage of instruments, and then instruments to be "issued for use." Monitoring of the sterilization process verifies the outcome of "sterilization" [8]. It includes equipment control, load control, biological monitoring, pack control, and exposure control. *Equipment control tests* determine the performance of the sterilizer with the use of Bowie-Dick test packs. *Load control* is the most important component of a sterilization monitoring program. It utilizes a biological indicator which should be placed in every cycle of a steam sterilizer [9]. *Pack control* uses chemical indicators for internal monitoring of packs and trays. Exposure control monitoring is a way for the sterilizer operators to know at a glance whether the packs have been exposed to the sterilization process. The most common process used is indicator tapes which undergo a color change when they have been exposed to the sterilant for details, refer Part 8.

- Quality assurance indicators in sterilization should be monitored, e.g., change in the color of indicator tape outside every surgical set, performing the Bowie and Dick test in every pre-vacuum steam sterilizer and once daily in the first unloaded cycle, change in the color of chemical indicator inside every instrument tray and on the ETO packing material, use of process challenge device (PCD) in ETO to ensure sterility of small lumen catheters, and weekly spore test reports from each and every type of sterilizer (Steam, ETO, Plasma).
- Use of "flash" sterilization has evolved over past years. However, these cycles should also be monitored properly [10].
- Microbiological air sampling in each theater should be done weekly.
- Clean and proper linen for both staff and patients during surgery is to be ensured.

An observational study published in 2011 [11] looked at the hand-hygiene practice in a medical center. The primary outcome observed was the hand-hygiene applications per staff per hour. In the 28 operations seen, an average of 0.14 hand-hygiene applications per hour per staff member were witnessed.

Monitoring of Infection Control Policy in Anesthesia

The environs of the operation theater are themselves a source for hospital-acquired infections. Anesthetic agents are associated with immune suppression; the staff in the OT touch patients frequently (shifting from the trolley, to the operating table and back to the trolley) [11]. Failure to apply hand hygiene will contaminate OT equipment and form a bank of pathogens which can infect all the patients who are operated in the theater.

The presence of pathogens has been shown on telephones, keyboards, and anesthesia machines [12–14].

Anesthesiologists perform invasive procedures such as tracheal intubation, arterial line insertions, and central venous catheter placements exposing patients to infection since the normal defense mechanisms are bypassed and neglected.

The infections related to anesthesia practice, within 72 h postoperatively, have been reported to be 3.4 % [15].

Anesthetic equipment is a potential source for transmission of infection [16]. Infection control policies regarding anesthesia equipment including anesthesia machines, face masks, airways, endotracheal tubes, laryngoscopes, and fiberoptic bronchoscopes should be in place. Monitoring with documentation of cleanliness standards should be done regularly. Policies regarding decontamination practices should be followed and audited for all reusable anesthetic equipment [17].

Certain invasive anesthetic procedures require optimum aseptic technique, e.g., insertion of central venous catheters and spinal, epidural, and caudal procedures. Care bundles, originally developed in the USA, systematically appraise these clinical procedures and help reduce catheter-related bacteremias [18].

The Infection Control Committee is responsible for making and monitoring compliance of policies.

Future

What does the future hold for adequate control of infection in operation theaters? The first thing that has to be considered is that infection control is not a static process; it is dynamic and dependent on several factors which in themselves are dynamic too. Despite stringent control on patient and doctor cleanliness and sterility of the operating environment and the equipment checks, all it takes is one careless individual with an infection to ruin the pristine confines of an operating field. Voice-activated machines are more effective as infection control devices.

Conclusion

Perioperative care of any surgical patient includes prevention of infection. The main preventive measures involve engineering and microbiological controls in the operating suite. Monitoring ventilation in the operating suite and microbiological monitoring of the ambient air, the surgical field, and instruments are essential for an infection-free outcome. Microbiological commissioning and monitoring of operating suites should adhere to national recommendations.

A regular checklist should be developed and followed, according to hospital protocol.

Infection control practice should be evidence based. Designing of new theater should have infection control in mind. Best practice is often based on expert opinion.

The anesthesiology motto fits well here "Eternal vigilance is the price of safety."

References

1. Working Party Report. Microbiological commissioning and monitoring of O.T. suites. J Hosp Infection. 2002;52:1–28.
2. Lidwell OM chair. Joint working party on ventilation in operating suites. Ventilation in operating suites. London MRC and DHSS. 1972.
3. NHS Estates. Health Building Note 26. Operating departments. 1991 ISBN 0113213859.
4. Noble WC. Dispersal of skin organisms. Br J Dermatol. 1975;93:477–85.
5. Whyte W, Hodgson R, Tinkler J. The importance of airborne bacterial contamination of wounds. J Hosp Infect. 1982;3:123–35.
6. NHS Estates. Ventilation in healthcare premises, Health Technical Memorandum, vol. 2025. London: HMSO; 1994.
7. Harte JA, Molinari JA. Sterilization procedures and monitoring. In: Molinari JA, Harte JA, editors. Cottone's practical infection control in dentistry. 3rd ed. Baltimore: Lippincott Williams and Wilkins; 2009. p. 148–70.

8. Nicolette LH. Infection prevention and control in the perioperative setting. In: Rothrock JC, editor. Alexander's care of the patient in surgery. 14th ed. St. Louis: Mosby; 2011. p. 67–8.
9. AORN. Recommended practices for sterilization in the perioperative practice setting. In: Perioperative standards and recommended practices. Denver: AORN; 2011. p. 429–85.
10. Larson D. Flash sterilization; exposing best practices in 2010. Healthcare Purchasing News. 2010:2–5.
11. Krediet AC, Kalkman CJ, Bonten MJ, Gigengack ACM, Barach P. Hand-hygiene practices in the operating theatre: an observational study. Br J Anaesth. 2011;107(4):553–8.
12. Jeske HC, Tiefenthaler W, Hohlrieder M, Hinterberger G, Benzer A. Bacterial contamination of anaesthetists' hands by personal mobile phone and fixed phone use in the operating theatre. Anaesthesia. 2007;62:904–6.
13. Fukada T, Iwakiri H, Ozaki M. Anaesthetists' role in computer key-board contamination in an operating room. J Hosp Infect. 2008;70:148–53.
14. Loftus RW, Koff MD, Burchman CC, et al. Transmission of patho-genic bacterial organisms in the anesthesia work area. Anesthesiology. 2008;109:399–407.
15. Hajjar J, Girard R. Surveillance of nosocomial infections related to anesthesia: a multicenter study. Ann Fr Anesth Reanim. 2000;19:47–53.
16. Association for the Advancement of Medical Instrumentation. Comprehensive guide to steam sterilization and sterility assurance in health care facilities. Arlington; ANSI/AAMI; ST79. 2010. p. 67–90.
17. Guidelines. Infection control in anaesthesia. Anaesthesia. 2008;63:1027–36.
18. Implement the central line bundle. http://www.ihi.org/IHI/Topics/CriticalCare/IntensiveCare/Changes/ImplementtheCentralLineBundle. Accessed 15 July 2008.

Monitoring of High-Risk Areas: Maternity Wards

Bhavna Anand and Kanwal Gujral

Obstetric population is vulnerable to infection in hospitals. Control and monitoring of infection in this population is a major area of concern. Impact of infection does occur on both the pregnant woman and her unborn or just born child. The importance of infection prevention and its impact was rightly described by Semmelwies in a natural experiment long time ago [1]. Since then there has been a major surge in this area to prevent maternity infection.

Sepsis accounts for about 15 % of global maternal mortality [2]. Maternity ward area is the prime area where infections are prevalent and where better results can be obtained if preventive and monitoring strategies are implemented. Maternity area includes a preparatory room, delivery area, recovery area (postpartum ward), and an attached observation nursery.

Sources of infection are as follows:

1. Endogenous
2. Exogenous

Most obstetric infections are polymicrobial, mainly due to endogenous maternal vaginal commensal flora which under specific circumstances become pathogens. They are represented by a mixture of anaerobes and gram-negative aerobic bacilli. Numbers of anaerobes outnumber aerobes and sexually transmitted infections also contribute to the flora [1]. The common organisms involved are included in Table 13.1.

Other organisms include Chlamydia and herpes simplex virus. Organisms causing neonatal sepsis are group B streptococcus, *E coli*. Prevention can be achieved by screening and treating vaginal colonization during pregnancy.

Exogenous factors include number of risk factors like the following:

1. Chronic maternal states – HIV, diabetes, bacterial vaginosis, syphilis, anemia
2. Obstetric factors – fever, prolonged rupture of membranes, prolonged catheterization, instrumental delivery, prolonged hospitalization, frequent internal examinations, intrauterine monitoring
3. Environmental factors – maternal age, socioeconomic status, maternal weight
4. Hospital malpractices – nonsegregation of infected and noninfected patients, infrequent surveillance of infection control program

Type of Infections

1. Surgical site infections (SSIs).
2. Postpartum endometritis – Caesarean section is associated with higher rate of PPE than vaginal delivery (10–20 %) [3].
3. Flare up of coexisting infection.
4. Chorioamnionitis.
5. Urinary tract infections.
6. Mastitis.
7. Early and late neonatal sepsis.

B. Anand (✉) • K. Gujral
Consultants, Institute of Obstetrics & Gynaecology,
Sir Ganga Ram Hospital, New Delhi, India
e-mail: bhavna027@rediffmail.com

C. Wattal and N. Khardori (eds.), *Hospital Infection Prevention: Principles & Practices*,
DOI 10.1007/978-81-322-1608-7_13, © Springer India 2014

Table 13.1 Common organisms involved in most obstetric infections

Anaerobes	Gram-positive aerobes	Gram-negative aerobes
Lactobacillus	*Staphylococcus* (coagulase negative)	*E. coli*
Peptostreptococcus	*Streptococci*	*Gardnerella vaginalis*
Bacteroides	*Staphylococcus aureus* (MRSA)	*Enterobacter*
Prevotella	*Enterococci*	*Klebsiella*
		Proteus mirabilis
		Ureaplasma
		Neisseria gonorrhoeae

Prevention and Monitoring of Infection

Essential components of infection prevention are practicing standard precautions (applied wherever contact with blood, body fluids, nonintact skin, mucous membranes, and secretion and excretion is expected) [4]. Obstetric population is exposed to invasive devices and procedure that carry a significant risk of infection transmission. Regular monitoring of simple measures as discussed below is mandatory in maternity wards.

1. *Hand hygiene* – Hand washing is one of the most important infection-preventing measures as recommended by WHO [5].
   (a) When to practice – Before and after handling blood or body fluids or direct contact with the patient, surgical scrub should be used for all invasive procedures.
   (b) Scrub time – Should not be less than 15–30 s. Hands should be properly dried after hand washing.
   (c) Agent used – CDC recommends use of plain water and soap for routine hand washing. Alcohol-containing hand disinfectants are an effective alternative. They have a rapid effect, are highly effective, and less time consuming; however, not much effect on spores like *Clostridium difficile* is noted [6].
   (d) Use of gloves – All staff should use gloves while working in the labor room as contact with patients or with body fluid is expected. Sterile latex gloves should be used for procedure involving skin or contact with nonintact mucous membranes. Gloves should be changed after contact with each patient. Hands must be washed when gloves are removed.
   (e) Compliance – Rarely exceed 45 % under best circumstances. This is largely due to unawareness and laziness among the staff.
2. *Use of masks, face shields, goggle, and gown* should be a practice in places where there is a risk of splash, spray of blood or body fluids.
3. *Sterilization and disinfection of instruments* – Sterilization is removing all living microorganisms, while disinfection is reducing the number of microorganisms. Different methods like heat and chemical are used for both sterilization and disinfection. Autoclaving is used for sterilizing delivery instruments. Hot water boiling cannot sterilize the instrument as bacterial spores resist boiling, but is an effective method of disinfection. The boiling should be done at least for 5 min when water returns to boiling. Chemical disinfection is another method of disinfection. Most common agent used is 2 % glutaraldehyde. Drawbacks are corrosive nature of agent used, variable effect on different organisms, and easy inactivation. Delivery sets should be autoclaved after using for each case. Equipments like neonatal kits should preferably be disposable. Regular surveillance to check proper sterilization should be done by sending regular swab cultures.
4. *Handling of sharp instruments* – should be handled with extreme caution and should be discarded in blue plastic waste bag [7].
5. *Handling of specimens* like placenta and others for pathological testing should be done carefully in appropriate container till it reaches laboratory; hands must be washed after handling specimens.
6. *Waste disposal* – Infectious and noninfectious wastes should be segregated and handled carefully. Labor room waste should be put and later

disposed in covered containers with special color coding and with minimal handling [7].

7. *Environmental cleaning* – All the rooms in the labor room should be properly ventilated to prevent airborne transmission. Patient should be advised to cover their mouths or nose while coughing and sneezing. All the hospital furniture including examination and delivery tables should be cleaned regularly. Floor should be cleaned daily with detergent. Any spill site should be cleaned with hypochlorite solution followed by detergent washing. Air-handling units should be cleaned at regular intervals and should provide 10–15 air changes/h. There should be restricted entry of visitors and relatives.

8. *Special precautions*

   (a) Preparation of patients going for delivery – Preparation of patients should be in a separate room from the delivery area. Cleaning should be done with savlon or chlorhexidine solution. Pubic hair should not be trimmed just prior to delivery as it increases the risk of infection.

   (b) Avoiding frequent internal examinations – This maneuver significantly reduces the incidence of postpartum endometritis and early neonatal sepsis. Frequent internal examinations should be avoided until necessary to prevent spread of ascending infections. Before every internal examination, proper antisepsis should be taken care of.

   (c) Care of breast, episiotomy, and cord – Breast should be regularly cleaned antenatally and before each feed postpartum. Episiotomy should be cared of by staff nurse twice to thrice a day and should be kept dry. Cord of baby should be cleaned with spirit at least thrice a day till it is completely dried.

   (d) Who should be isolated – Provision of a separate septic labor room should be there in every maternity ward to keep potentially infectious patients like patients with fever, gastroenteritis, other infectious diseases, puerperal infection, breast infection, or infectious newborn.

   (e) High-risk cases

      1. Preterm premature rupture of membranes (PPROM) – PPROM occurs in 3 % of all pregnancies and 30 % of all preterm labors. Identification, diagnosis, antibiotics, and timely delivery can reduce serious risk of intra-amniotic infections and neonatal sepsis.

      2. Chronic infection – Isolation of mothers with hepatitis B, hepatitis C, HIV, and herpes simplex viral infection. They should be cared of in isolation with immunized staff. Their waste should be considered as infectious and disposed of separately. The patients should be monitored aggressively with restricted internal monitoring. Immunization/ART should be given to newborn to prevent vertical transmission.

      3. GBS prophylaxis – GBS, Group B streptococcus (*Streptococcus agalactiae*) is the most frequent cause of severe early onset neonatal sepsis (at less than 7 days of birth) [8]. The preventive strategies include clear delivery practices and intrapartum antibiotic prophylaxis (IAP). Indications for offering GBS-specific IAP are as follows: 1. previous baby with invasive GBS infection, 2. GBS bacteriuria in the current pregnancy, 3. vaginal swab positive for GBS in current pregnancy, 4. pyrexia (>38 °C in labor), and 5. chorioamnionitis.

IAP for GBS is not necessary if delivery occurs by pre-labor lower segment section with intact membranes [8].

9. *Surveillance* – Regular auditing and surveillance of all the preventive strategies is the key to achieve success in its implementation. Key components of a surveillance program in a maternity ward are as follows:

   1. Provision of a special team comprising of doctors, staff nurse, and microbiologist for weekly random rounds and observe clean practices among staff

   2. Regular teaching and training of all the new and old staff about infection prevention measures

   3. Detail review of patients admitting with complaints of wound discharge, episiotomy

gaping, neonatal sepsis, fever, or for reexploration
4. Testing of staff for carrier stated of chronic diseases specially MRSA

Conclusion

To conclude, a majority of labor room infections can be prevented by implementation of clean practices in the labor room.

References

1. Mayhall CG, editor. Hospital epidemiology and infection control. 4th ed. Philadelphia: Lippincott Williams & Wilkins; 2011. p. 787–94.
2. Park K. Text book of preventive and social medicine. 21st ed. Jabalpur: Banarsidas Bhanot; 2011. p. 514–17.
3. Kluytmans JAJW. Infection control in obstetrics. In: Wenzel R, Bearman G, Brewer T, Butzier JP, editors. Guide to infection control in the hospital. 4th ed. Boston: International Society of Infectious Diseases; 2008. p. 219–22.
4. Garner JS. Guideline for isolation precautions in hospitals. The Hospital Infection Control Practices Advisory Committee. Infect Control Hosp Epidemiol. 1996;17(1):53–80.
5. Pittet D, Allegranzi B, Sax H, Dharan S, Pessoa-Silva CL, Donaldson L, Boyce JM. Evidence-based model for hand transmission during patient care and the role of improved practices. Lancet Infect Dis. 2006;6(10):641–52.
6. Guidelines on infection control practice in clinic and maternity homes. www.info.gov.hk/aids/pdf/916.pdf
7. Park K. Text Book of preventive and social medicine. 21st ed. Jabalpur: Banarsidas Bhanot; 2011. p. 730–34.
8. The prevention of early onset neonatal Group B streptococcal disease, RCOG Green top guidelines no. 36. 2nd ed. Available at: http://www.rcog.org.uk/guidelines. Accessed on 28 Dec 2012.

Monitoring of High-Risk Areas: Cancer Wards

14

Jeewan Garg and Anupam Sachdeva

Infection continues to be the foremost cause of morbidity and mortality in patients undergoing antineoplastic chemotherapy. Despite improved diagnostic tools, better understanding of infectious etiologies, and the advent of several new antimicrobials, infections continue to be a major problem [1]. Cancer patients suffer from host immune system defects and anatomic barrier disruption that predispose them to infections. Understanding the different risk factors in the individual patient is necessary to implement the appropriate preventive strategies.

Factors that predispose to infectious diseases include those related to the underlying malignancy and treatment-related immunosuppression. Neutropenia is the most common risk factor for infection in cancer patients. The lack of granulocytes facilitates bacterial and fungal infections and blunts the inflammatory response, allowing infections to progress much faster. Neutropenia, asplenia, high-dose corticosteroids, and lymphocyte-depleting agents represent different forms of immunocompromise that increases the risk of different kinds of infection. Selected host defense defects encountered in patients with cancer are presented in Table 14.1 [2].

The mucosal linings of the gastrointestinal, respiratory, and genitourinary tracts constitute the first line of host defense against a variety of pathogens. Besides the physical barrier, mucosal epithelial cells secrete a variety of antimicrobial peptides, including lactoferrin, lysozyme, phospholipase A2, and defensins. Chemotherapy and radiation therapy impair mucosal immunity at several different levels. When the physical protective barrier conferred by the epithelial lining is compromised, local flora may invade, and bacteremia and candidemia may result. Host anatomic barrier disruption and their associated infectious pathogens are presented in Table 14.2 [3].

Major Factors Predisposing Cancer Patients to Develop Infections Are as Follows

1. The type of cancer, especially one which has its origins in the blood/immune system.
2. The depth and duration of immunosuppression (e.g., neutropenia and lymphopenia) associated with the cancer and/or its treatment.
3. Other blood parameters such as anemia, which affect performance status and thrombocytopenia, which may be associated with bleeding/bruising, predisposing to infection.
4. The toxicity of the cancer treatment and especially mucosal damage of the gastrointestinal tract which facilitates invasion by gut microbes.
5. Breaks in skin integrity whether spontaneous or iatrogenic, i.e., associated with medical interventions. These breaks in skin facilitate the entry of native and hospital-acquired organisms.

J. Garg
Department of Hematology, Sir Ganga Ram Hospital, New Delhi, India

A. Sachdeva (✉)
Institute of Child Health, Sir Ganga Ram Hospital, New Delhi, India
e-mail: anupamace@yahoo.co.in

Table 14.1 Risk factors and associated infections in cancer patients

Risk factors	Infection	Infection-predisposing host defects
Malignancy-related factors		
Hematologic malignancies		
Myelodysplastic syndrome and acute leukemia	Bacteria, viruses, and fungi	Prolonged neutropenia
Chronic lymphocytic leukemia	Encapsulated bacteria	Hypogammaglobulinemia, abnormal cell-mediated immunity
Multiple myeloma	Encapsulated bacteria	Impaired B-cell immunity, hypogammaglobulinemia
Hairy cell leukemia	Mycobacteria, herpes viruses	Neutropenia, defective T-cell immunity
Hodgkin's lymphoma	Mycobacteria, herpes viruses	Defective T-cell immunity
Adult T-cell lymphoma/leukemia	*Pneumocystis jiroveci, Cryptococcus neoformans,* cytomegalovirus, *Strongyloides stercoralis*	Defective T-cell immunity
Solid tumors		
Endobronchial tumors	Postobstructive pneumonia	Mechanical obstruction
Colon carcinoma	*Streptococcal bacteremia*	Mechanical disruption
	Clostridium bacteremia	
Hepatobiliary tumors	Bacterial infection with enteric organisms	Mechanical obstruction plus abnormal liver function if underlying cirrhosis
Head and neck cancer	Infections with oral flora and anaerobes	Mechanical disruption
Genitourinary tumors	Gram-negative bacilli, *Enterococcus* sp.	Related to obstruction
Treatment-related factors		
Neutropenia	Bacterial and fungal infections	
Mucositis	Bacterial infections caused by oral and enteric flora, candidiasis	
Corticosteroids	Bacteria, *Pneumocystis jiroveci, Cryptococcus neoformans,* molds, herpes viruses	Impaired phagocytic function and cell-mediated immunity, decrease signs and symptoms of inflammation
Nucleoside analogues (e.g., fludarabine)	Bacteria, *P. jiroveci, C. neoformans,* herpes viruses	Defective T-cell immunity by T-cell depletion
Alemtuzumab	Opportunistic and non-opportunistic infections, including bacteria, viruses (e.g., CMV, VZV), *P. jiroveci,* and fungi	Broad defect in host defense involving depletion of T, B, and NK cells and monocytes, occasional neutropenia
Rituximab	Bacterial infections, VZV, *P. jiroveci*	Impaired B-cell immunity
Daclizumab	Bacterial sepsis	Infections in the setting of steroid-refractory GVHD
Antibodies inhibiting cytokine signaling (e.g., infliximab)	Bacterial infections, tuberculosis, and other mycobacterial infections, mold infections in GVHD	Suppression of inflammation may allow infections to progress undetected
Calcineurin inhibitors	*Pneumocystis jiroveci,* VZV	Defective T-cell immunity
Radiation therapy	Local and systemic bacterial infections, mucosal candidiasis and HSV infection	Damages mucosal surfaces, marrow suppression

CMV cytomegalovirus, *VZV* varicella-zoster virus, *NK* natural killer, *GVHD* graft-versus-host disease, *HSV* herpes simplex virus

Table 14.2 Anatomic barrier disruption and associated pathogens

Anatomic disruption	Pathogen categories
Oral cavity (mucositis)	α-Hemolytic streptococci, oral anaerobes
	Candida species
	Herpes simplex virus
Esophagus	Candida species
	Herpes simplex virus, cytomegalovirus
Lower gastrointestinal tract	Enterococcus, gram-negative enteric organisms
	Anaerobes (Bacteroides fragilis, Clostridium perfringens)
	Candida species
	Strongyloides stercoralis
Skin (IV catheter)	Gram-positive staphylococci and streptococci, Corynebacteria, Bacillus
	Atypical mycobacteria
Urinary tract	Enterococcus
	Gram-negative enteric organisms
	Candida species
Splenectomy	Encapsulated organisms: S. pneumoniae, H. influenzae, Neisseria meningitidis
	Capnocytophaga canimorsus
	Salmonella (especially sickle cell disease)
	Babesia

6. The use of long-term vascular catheters such as Hickman lines is a risk factor for catheter-associated bloodstream infection. Prolonged venous access for the administration of chemotherapy is required in large numbers of cancer patients.

7. Coexisting medical conditions, e.g., chronic renal failure and diabetes mellitus.

8. The performance status (activity level) of the individual, e.g., fully active versus bed confined.

9. Suboptimal physical facilities within which care is delivered with particular reference to cross infection and the sharing of toilet facilities.

10. The level of adherence by healthcare staff to guidelines on infection prevention and control in hospitals and elsewhere such as hospices, while looking after such a vulnerable population.

11. The availability of adequate support such as transfusion, clinical nutrition, hospice care, physiotherapy, and psychological support which serve to improve performance status and to keep the patient out of hospital when that is possible during cancer treatment.

Monitoring of Cancer Wards

Monitoring of wards for prevention and control of infection in most hospitals is done by infection control team. An infection control program should be overseen by infection control team chaired by an infectious disease physician and consisting of staff representing departments throughout the facility, such as nursing, pharmacy, clinical microbiology, central sterilization services, housekeeping, maintenance, food services, and laundry services. Among the responsibilities of an infection control team are to do the following:

- Conduct surveillance of nosocomial infections
- Develop policies regarding prevention and control of infection
- Ensure adherence to standards for environmental services
- Establish a program to monitor and evaluate antimicrobial therapy
- Obtain appropriate microbiologic specimens when infection is suspected or present
- Provide education to healthcare personnel about adherence to infection control policies
- Develop guidelines for outbreak preparedness

The infection control team develops a system for identifying, reporting, analyzing, investigating, and controlling hospital-acquired infections. The infection control team also develops and implements preventive and corrective programs in specific situations where infection hazards exist. The infection control team does the following:

- Establishes a system for monitoring bacterial resistance and antibiotic usage, including the quantity and patterns of use, and provides feedback of results to prescribers
- Develops and regularly update guidelines for antimicrobial treatment and prophylaxis

- Conducts surveillance through open communication with the nursing staff and physicians and meticulous review of patient records and microbiology results
- Takes culture swabs from environmental surfaces and air sampling plates periodically from high-risk areas like bone marrow transplant units
- Monitors ward housekeepers to make sure that standards of cleaning and disinfection of environmental surfaces, beds, bedrails, bedside equipment, and other frequently touched surfaces are achieved
- Monitors catering to make sure that all food is prepared in a safe and clean way
- Monitors laundry to make sure that all linen is cleaned correctly to minimize infection
- Monitors estate and building services to make sure that any building work is carried out with the minimum of dust and dirt
- Ensures that potable water testing for bacterial cultures carried out routinely from all patient care units and hospital kitchen
- Monitors hospital decontamination unit to make sure that high standards are maintained
  For details, see Chap. 4

Prevention of Infections

Infections in cancer patients may be prevented by several different and complementary strategies such as the following:

1. The simplest and most effective means of preventing transmission of infection has proven to be meticulous hand washing by physicians, nurses, and others who are in close contact with patients [4].
2. Avoid hospitalization when possible and if appropriate [5].
3. Avoid overcrowding and unnecessary through traffic in the cancer and bone marrow transplant wards.
4. Consider protective isolation for high-risk patients [5]. All immunosuppressed or contagious patients should be isolated in separate rooms. When a single room is not available, patients colonized or infected with the same

microorganisms may be nursed together in a designated area or ward (cohort nursing).
5. *Barrier Nursing*: The aim is to erect a barrier to the passage of infectious pathogenic organisms between the immunosuppressed or contagious patient and other patients and staff in the hospital and hence to the outside world. The nurses, attending consultants, and any visitors must wear gown, mask, cap, shoe cover, and sometimes gloves, and they must observe strict rules that minimize the risk of passing on infectious agents.
6. Use of granulocyte colony-stimulating factors (GCSFs) to shorten the duration of neutropenia [5].
7. Use immunosuppressive drugs judiciously.
8. Avoid invasive procedures, except when absolutely necessary, and remove venous lines as soon as possible [5]. Strict aseptic techniques should be maintained when manipulating intravascular catheter systems.
9. Provide prompt treatment of prior active sites of infection.
10. Monitor serological tests and clinical course in patients with known history of infection exposure (such as hepatitis B, tuberculosis), and consider prophylactic drugs [5].
11. Consider prophylactic antimicrobials in high-risk patients [5].
12. Patients with cancer should be vaccinated with recommended vaccines, which are primarily focused on preventing acquisition of community-acquired infections.
13. A cooked-food diet that excludes fresh fruits and vegetables and non-processed dairy products during periods of neutropenia is advocated [6, 7].
14. Ensure proper construction and frequent upkeep of ventilation systems. Laminar airflow rooms and high-efficiency particulate air (HEPA) filtration are important for certain high-risk patients, such as those undergoing bone marrow transplant, as their use has decreased the incidence of Aspergillus infections [8].
15. Provide serial monitoring of hospital water supply and of cooling and heating systems for microbial contamination [5].

16. Patients, their families, and all healthcare workers need to be educated on simple measures that can minimize infection, including standard precautions and important aspects of personal and environmental hygiene. The care of central venous lines, skin care, and oral and perineal hygiene are areas of particular concern.

17. National surveillance strategies should collect data on infections in cancer patients.

Antimicrobials Prophylaxis

The key to antimicrobial prophylaxis is to know the spectrum of infection-causing pathogens at the individual clinical center. Antimicrobial prophylaxis should be provided to high-risk patients.

Antibacterial Prophylaxis

Trimethoprim-sulfamethoxazole (TMP-SMZ) has been used for many years for prophylaxis against bacterial infections. Initial studies using this drug showed its efficacy in preventing *Pneumocystis jiroveci* [9]. Later studies demonstrated its benefit in reducing the incidence of bacterial infections in patients with hematologic malignancies [10]. Quinolone-based prophylaxis has been successful in reducing the risk of aerobic gram-negative infections in neutropenic patients who undergo cytotoxic chemotherapy for acute leukemia and bone marrow transplantation [11, 12]. However, emergence of secondary resistance remains a problem.

Antifungal Prophylaxis

Risk factors for fungal infections in cancer patients include prolonged and profound neutropenia, immunosuppressive therapy, use of broad-spectrum antibiotics, use of parenteral nutrition, and use of indwelling vascular devices. Preventive efforts toward the reduction of fungal infections in these patients have focused primarily on Candida and Aspergillus species, as they have traditionally been the most common causes of fungal disease in immunocompromised patients [13]. In several randomized trials in patients with leukemia and patients who were undergoing allogeneic stem cell transplantation, fluconazole prophylaxis at a dosage of 400 mg/day reduced the incidence of superficial and invasive candidal infections, except those caused by *C. krusei* [14, 15].

Antiviral Prophylaxis

Acquisition of opportunistic viral disease may occur by primary infection or by reactivation of latent infection. Herpes viruses, including CMV, VZV, and HSV-1 and -2, are by far the most common infection-causing viruses. Administration of oral or intravenous acyclovir prevents HSV reactivation (gingivostomatitis, esophagitis) in patients who are receiving intensive chemotherapy for acute leukemia or bone marrow transplantation [16, 17].

Augmentation of Host Defenses

Despite several advances in antimicrobial prophylaxis, efforts to prevent infections in immunocompromised patients with cancer have been disappointing. One of the possible ways to reduce infection risk may be to booster the immune status of the host. There are several ways of boosting the immune status of the host such as use of granulocyte colony-stimulating factors (GCSFs) and active and passive immunization. Neutropenia continues to be the most significant dose-limiting toxicity of systemic chemotherapy. Discovery of the recombinant human growth factors has been revolutionary in the management of chemotherapy-induced neutropenia [5].

References

1. Bodey GP. Managing infections in the immunocompromised patient. Clin Infect Dis. 2005;40 Suppl 4:S239.

2. Gea-Banacloche JC, Palmore T, Walsh TJ, Holland SM, Segal BH. Infections in the cancer patient. In: DeVita VT, Lawrence TS, Rosenberg SA, editors. Principles & practice of oncology. 8th ed. Philadelphia: Lippincott Williams & Wilkins; 2008. p. 2569–616.

3. Young JH, Weisdorf DJ. Clinical approach to infections in the compromised host. In: Hoffman R, Benz EJ, Shattil SJ, Furie B, Silberstein LE, McGlave P, et al., editors. Hematology: basic principles and practice. 5th ed. Philadelphia: Churchill Livingstone Elsevier; 2009. p. 1243–88.

4. Larson EL. APIC guideline for hand washing and hand antisepsis in health care settings. Am J Infect Control. 1995;23:251–69.

5. Vusirikala M. Supportive care in hematologic malignancies. In: Greer JP, Foerster J, Rodgers GM, Paraskevas F, Glader B, Arber DA, et al., editors. Wintrobe's clinical hematology. 12th ed. Philadelphia: Lippincott Williams & Wilkins; 2009. p. 1747–90.

6. DeMille D, Deming P, Lupinacci P, et al. The effect of the neutropenic diet in the outpatient setting: a pilot study. Oncol Nurs Forum. 2006;33:337–43.

7. Wilson BJ. Dietary recommendations for neutropenic patients. Semin Oncol Nurs. 2002;18:44–9.

8. Hahn T, Cummings KM, Michalek AM, et al. Efficacy of high-efficiency particulate air filtration in preventing aspergillosis in immunocompromised patients with hematologic malignancies. Infect Control Hosp Epidemiol. 2002;23:525–31.

9. Hughes WT, Rivera GK, Schell MJ, et al. Successful intermittent chemoprophylaxis for Pneumocystis carinii pneumonitis. N Engl J Med. 1987; 316:1627–32.

10. De Pauw BE, Novakova IR, Ubachs E, et al. Co-trimoxazole in patients with haematological malignancies: a review of 10-years' clinical experience. Curr Med Res Opin. 1988;11:64–72.

11. Engels EA, Lau J, Barza M. Efficacy of quinolone prophylaxis in neutropenic cancer patients: a meta-analysis. J Clin Oncol. 1998;16:1179–87.

12. Imran H, Tlvejeh IM, Arndt CA, et al. Fluoroquinolone prophylaxis in patients with neutropenia: a meta-analysis of randomized placebo-controlled trials. Eur J Clin Microbiol Infect Dis. 2008;27:53–63.

13. Bow EJ, Laverdiere M, Lussier N, et al. Antifungal prophylaxis for severely neutropenic chemotherapy recipients: a meta analysis of randomized-controlled clinical trials. Cancer. 2002;94:3230–46.

14. Winston DJ, Chandrasekar PH, Lazarus HM, et al. Fluconazole prophylaxis of fungal infections in patients with acute leukemia. Results of a randomized, placebo-controlled, double-blind, multicenter trial. Ann Intern Med. 1993;118:495–503.

15. Robenshtok E, Gafter-Gvili A, Goldberg E, et al. Antifungal prophylaxis in cancer patients after chemotherapy or hematopoietic stem-cell transplantation: systematic review and meta-analysis. J Clin Oncol. 2007;25:5471–89.

16. Saral R, Ambinder RF, Burns WH, et al. Acyclovir prophylaxis against herpes simplex virus infection in patients with leukemia. A randomized, double-blind, placebo-controlled study. Ann Intern Med. 1983;99:773–6.

17. Selby PJ, Powles RL, Easton D, et al. The prophylactic role of intravenous and long term oral acyclovir after allogeneic bone marrow transplantation. Br J Cancer. 1989;59:434–8.

Monitoring of High-Risk Areas: Dialysis Units

15

Ashwini Gupta

Patients having chronic kidney disease (CKD) are more susceptible to a wide range of infections due to their unique position whereby they have more chances of exposure to various pathogens due to decreased immune defenses and increased interventions especially in patients on hemodialysis. According to Indian CKD registry data, of all the end-stage renal disease (ESRD) patients receiving any dialysis, more than 86 % are on maintenance hemodialysis [1].

Maintenance hemodialysis patients are at increased risk for infection because of defective immunity, and the process involves a vascular access use in environment where opportunities for transmission of infectious agents exist [2]. Even otherwise, ESRD patients are more prone to infections as the population undergoing hemodialysis is increasingly becoming more elderly. In this scenario, it becomes all the more imperative on the concerned nephrologist to understand the risks of infection in dialysis patients and prevent them as far as possible.

Infections in dialysis patients may involve four components:

I. Infections related to hemodialysis system
II. Infections related to vascular access
III. Infections unique to dialysis unit
IV. Other infections

A. Gupta, M.D. (✉)
Department of Nephrology, Sir Ganga Ram Hospital, New Delhi, India
e-mail: ashwani_gupta@yahoo.com

Infections Related to Hemodialysis System

Bacterial Infections

The aqueous environments associated with hemodialysis equipment can act as a growth medium for multiplication and proliferation of gram-negative bacteria leading to massive organism burden which might cause septicemia or endotoxemia in patients. These bacteria can form biofilms (glycocalyces) on the surface of hemodialysis equipment which are almost impossible to eradicate [3]. Infection control strategies in dialysis units are formed with target of keeping the concentration of organism at an acceptable low level.

Although gram-negative bacteria and nontuberculous mycobacteria like *Mycobacterium avium*, *M. fortuitum*, *M. intracellulare*, *M. kansasii*, and M. scrofulaceum are the commoner organisms present in dialysis system, virtually any organism that can grow in water is a threat [4].

When treated water is mixed with dialysis concentrate, the resulting dialysis fluid is a balanced salt solution and growth medium which is nutrient rich for proliferation of organisms. Bacterial growth in water used for hemodialysis depends on the following:

1. The source of water
2. The water treatment system
3. The distribution system
4. The dialysis machine
5. The disinfection method

Water used in dialysis unit is obtained from the community water supply, and it can become contaminated with bacteria and endotoxins. The main microbes contaminating dialysis water include bacteria (gram-negative bacteria and nontuberculous mycobacteria) [3]. However, contamination with fungi and blue green algae besides many viruses like hepatitis, poliomyelitis may also take place [5]. Endotoxins are important in causing pyrogenic reactions during hemodialysis.

A water treatment system treats the tap water to produce a purified form of water which is chemically adequate and has an acceptable level of microbes. The components in a typical water treatment plant include the following:

1. Prefilters (depth filters)
2. Water softener
3. Carbon tanks (adsorption tanks)
4. Particulate filter
5. Reverse osmosis unit
6. Deionization unit
7. Storage tank
8. Ultrafilter

As the incoming tap water passes through the system components, it becomes more chemically pure, but the level of microbial contamination increases, emphasizing the importance of ultrafiltration and reverse osmosis.

In the water treatment plant, there may be contamination at level of initial filtration (depth filter) which filters bacteria, but do not remove them, hence, over a period of time, may become saturated with bacteria and lead to bacterial growth through the filter. Hence, they need to be changed regularly. Softeners in water treatment plant remove cations and anions, but they are also a source of bacteria and endotoxins, needing to be changed regularly. Carbon tanks remove chlorine/chloramines and organic substances, but they can also be contaminated with bacteria. Reverse osmosis units used in water treatment plants remove bacteria, endotoxins, and other chemicals. They are required to be cleaned regularly.

Ultraviolet irradiation kills most bacteria, but there is a possibility of UV-resistant pathogens remaining post-UV which has to be kept in mind. Ultrafilter used after reverse osmosis further removes bacteria and endotoxins, but they are also needed to be changed regularly.

Various factors of water distribution system also increase risk of colonization of bacteria and biofilm formation: large diameters and long length of distribution pipes, material of pipes used in system, and dead ends in system and storage tanks. The large diameter of pipes and longer length makes the pipes vulnerable for biofilm formation by increasing area for colonization. Dead ends in the distribution network also keep stagnant water which may increase colonization. So, the distribution system should not have dead ends, and the outlets to the dialysis machines should have as short a path as feasible to reduce dead space and thereby the chances of microbial colonization and biofilm formation. The storage tank also increases the surface area for colonization. It is desired to have a storage tank with conical base so that it can be drained completely. The storage tanks should be routinely cleaned, disinfected, and drained. If a biofilm is formed, it may require strong oxidizers or even scrubbing of the inner surface of the tank to remove it. From a storage tank, the water should pass through an ultrafilter before reaching the distribution system.

Routine disinfection of the water supply and distribution network should be performed regularly, once a month at least [12]. The minimum standards needed for the purity of water used to prepare dialysis solution are given by various authorities like AAMI (Advancement of Medical Instrumentation) as well as European Dialysis and Transplant Association (Table 15.1) [6, 11]. Current AAMI recommendations are that product water used to prepare dialysis solution, and the resultant dialysis solution, should contain <200 colony-forming units (CFU)/mL of bacteria and <2.0 endotoxin units (EU)/mL of endotoxin [11]. AAMI recommends action at >50 CFU/ml and >1 EU/ml. The maximum values recommended by EDTA are <100 CFU/mL and <0.25 EU/mL, respectively [6]. For ultrapure dialysate, AAMI recommends <0.1 CFU/ml and <0.03 EU/ml. There is a case of close surveillance by the Hospital Infection Control Committee in this matter.

Table 15.1 Standards for quality of dialysis water and dialysis fluid

Standard	Water		Dialysis fluid	
	Viable counts (CFU/ml)	Endotoxin	Viable counts (CFU/ml)	Endotoxin
European Dialysis and Transplant Association (EDTA) [6]	<100	<0.25 EU/ml	<100	<0.25 EU/ml
German Dialysis Standard (hygiene guideline) [7]	<100	<0.25 EU/ml	<100	<0.25 EU/ml
Japanese Society for Dialysis Therapy [8]	<100	<0.05 EU/ml	<100	<0.05 EU/ml
Swedish pharmacopoeia [9]	<100	<0.25 IU/ml	<100	<0.25 IU/ml
Canadian Standards Association (CSA) [10]	<100	<2 EU/ml	<100	<2 EU/ml
AAMI Standards (USA) [11]	≤200	<2 EU/ml	≤200	<2 EU/ml

It should be ensured that the disinfectant remains for adequate time in the distribution network and is not drained off before the minimum period required to achieve adequate disinfection. The distribution systems should be designed with all taps at equal elevation and at the highest point of the system to prevent the disinfectant from draining off. The system should be free of rough joints, dead-end pipes, and taps as the fluid trapped in such stagnant areas can serve as reservoirs for bacteria and fungi that later contaminate the rest of the distribution system [13].

Disinfection of dialysis systems can be done using sodium hypochlorite 1 %, 4 % formaldehyde, hydrogen peroxide, glutaraldehyde, peracetic acids, ozone, and hot-water pasteurization. Sodium hypochlorite solutions are convenient and effective in most parts of the dialysis system. Usually, the dialysis machine is disinfected using sodium hypochlorite at start of the dialysis session as chlorine is corrosive and needs to be rinsed out of system after short period of time, so it cannot be kept overnight [14]. Other disinfectants like peroxyacetate, hydrogen peroxide, and glutaraldehyde are used at the end of the day for disinfection [15]. Hot-water disinfection (pasteurization) has also been used in some dialysis systems whereby water is heated to >80 °C and passed through the system. It is a very satisfactory mode for disinfection.

Samples of source water, water obtained from critical points in the water treatment system and distribution network, product water, dialysate,

and bicarbonate solution must be cultured at least once a month to ensure that bacterial contamination is compliant to AAMI standards.

Water samples should be collected from a source as close as possible to where water enters the dialysate proportioning unit, usually the tap (not from that hose connecting the tap to the dialysis machine) at the dialysis station. Samples should also be collected whenever any modifications or maintenance is done to the water treatment and distribution systems. Dialysate samples should be collected during or at the end of the dialysis treatment from a source close to where the dialysis fluid either enters or leaves the dialyzer. Samples of water and dialysate should also be collected when pyrogenic reactions are suspected. Water used to prepare disinfectant and rinse dialyzers should also be assayed monthly if the dialysis center is reusing dialyzers.

Specimens should be assayed within 30 min of collection or, if being stored, to be refrigerated at 4 °C and must be assayed within 24 h of collection. Conventional laboratory methods such as the pour plate, spread plate, or membrane filter technique can be used. Calibrated loops should not be used because they sample a small volume and are inaccurate. Trypticase soy agar (soybean casein digest agar) should be used for growth. The assay should be quantitative, not qualitative, and a standard technique should be used. Colonies should be counted after 48 h of incubation at 36 °C [16]. Total viable counts are the objective of plate counts. Endotoxin testing should be conducted using either Limulus amebocyte lysate assay either Gel-clot method or one of the kinetic methods. In an outbreak investigation, the assay methods may need to be both qualitative and quantitative; also detection of nontuberculous mycobacteria and in some cases fungi in water or dialysate may be desirable. In such instances plates should be incubated for 5–14 days at both 36 °C and 28 °C–30 °C.

Pyrogen Reactions

Pyrogen reactions can be defined as objective chills (visible rigors) or fever (temperature >37.8 °C [100 °F]) or both in a patient who was afebrile and had no signs or symptoms of an infection before the start of the dialysis treatment session [17]. These are usually caused by gram-negative bacteria contaminating the dialysis water or components of the dialysis system. These may start within 2–5 h of initiation of dialysis. They may be associated with headache, nausea, vomiting, body aches, hypotension, and myalgia. Pyrogenic reactions can occur without bacteria; because presenting signs and symptoms cannot differentiate bacteremia from pyrogenic reactions, blood cultures are necessary. Pyrogenic reactions can result from passage of bacterial endotoxin (lipopolysaccharide [LPS]) or other substances in the dialysate across the dialyzer membrane or the transmembrane stimulation of cytokine production in the patient's blood by endotoxin in the dialysate. Endotoxin can also enter directly into the blood stream with fluids that are contaminated with gram-negative bacteria.

The signs and symptoms of pyrogenic reactions without bacteremia generally subside within a few hours after the dialysis has been stopped. If gram-negative sepsis is associated, fever and chills may persist, and hypotension is more refractory to therapy.

When a pyrogenic reaction occurs, a careful physical examination of the patient should be done to rule out other causes of chills and fever (e.g., pneumonia, vascular access infection, urinary tract infection). Investigations including blood cultures, chest x-ray, and urine culture should be done. A sample of the dialysate from the dialyzer (downstream side) should also be taken for quantitative and qualitative microbiological culture.

Infections Related to Vascular Access

Vascular access remains a major area of concern as far as infections in hemodialysis patients are concerned. Vascular access site infections are particularly important because they can cause disseminated bacteremia or loss of the vascular access. They may arise either from any of the following:
1. Migration of the patient's own skin flora onto the outer catheter surface
2. Contamination of the catheter connectors
3. Lumen contamination during dialysis
4. Infused solutions
5. Colonization of catheters from more remote sites during bacteremia

Vascular access infections may present with redness, tenderness, swelling, warmth, localized pus discharge, or ulcerations [18, 19].

In the CDC surveillance project, the initial reported rates of access-associated bacteremia per 100 patient months were 1.8 overall and varied by access type: 0.25 for fistulas, 0.53 for grafts, 4.8 for permanent (tunneled, cuffed) catheters, and 8.7 for temporary (nontunneled, noncuffed) catheters [19]. Another analysis of data revealed that the overall vascular access infection rate was 3.1 per 100 patient months and varied from 0.6 for fistulas to 10.1 for temporary catheters [20].

Organisms causing vascular access infections include *Staphylococcus aureus* (32–53 % of cases), coagulase-negative staphylococci (20–32 % of cases), gram-negative bacilli (10–18 %), other gram-positive cocci (including enterococci; 10–12 %), and fungi (<1 %) [19, 21]. The proportion of infections caused by *S. aureus* is higher among patients with fistulas or grafts, and the proportion caused by coagulase-negative staphylococci is higher among patients dialyzed through catheters. Risk for infection depends on the type of vascular access (maximum for catheter, minimum for arteriovenous fistulas, and intermediate for arteriovenous graft) [20, 21]. A variety of other risk factors influence access site infection like diabetes, poor hygiene, old age, hematoma formation, poor needle insertion technique, recent vascular surgery, trauma or hematoma over the access site, immunosuppression, intravenous drug abuse, and iron overload [20–22].

Based on relative risk of both infectious and noninfectious complications, use of AV fistulas is promoted over the use of hemodialysis catheters. It is recommended to have no more than 10 % of patients maintained with permanent catheter-based hemodialysis treatment [23, 24]. To minimize infectious complications, patients should be referred early for creation vascular access, thereby decreasing the time dialyzed through a temporary catheter. Additionally, catheters should be used only in patients for whom a permanent access is impossible. These infections can be minimized by maintaining complete asepsis while inserting and handling catheters, minimizing the duration of catheter use, and avoiding use of uncuffed femoral catheters as far as possible.

Recommendations for preventing hemodialysis catheter-associated infections include [23–26] the following:

1. Not using antimicrobial prophylaxis before insertion or during use of the catheter
2. Not routinely replacing the catheter
3. Using sterile technique (cap, mask, sterile gown, large sterile drapes, and gloves) during catheter insertion
4. Limiting use of noncuffed catheters to 3–4 weeks
5. Using the catheter solely for hemodialysis unless there is no other alternative
6. Restricting catheter manipulation and dressing changes to trained personnel
7. Replacing catheter site dressing at each dialysis session or if damp, loose, or soiled
8. Disinfecting skin before catheter insertion and dressing changes

Prophylactic local antibiotics like mupirocin ointment at the catheter exit site may be used in documented S. aureus carriers to lower colonization. Povidone ointment, polysporin ointment, and topical honey also have been used to reduce the risk of central venous catheter-associated bacteremia. Antimicrobial catheter lock solutions reduce catheter-related bloodstream infections although CDC does not recommend the routine use of antimicrobial lock solutions for hemodialysis catheters because antimicrobial use can lead to antimicrobial resistance.

In hemodialysis patients, the Infectious Disease Society of America has recommended treatment with nasal mupirocin in documented S. aureus carriers who have catheter-related blood stream infection with S. aureus and continue to need a hemodialysis catheter [27, 28]. Otherwise the routine use of nasal mupirocin in patients with hemodialysis catheters is not recommended by either CDC or the National Kidney Foundation [23, 25].

Infections Unique to the Dialysis Unit

Transmission of infections in hemodialysis units may occur by spread from patient to patient, use of infected blood, or breach of universal precautions. These include hepatitis B virus (HBV) and hepatitis C virus (HCV) infections.

Prevalence of hepatitis B and C in dialysis units can be controlled by following strict yet simple steps like mandatory hepatitis B vaccination in all CKD patients, screening all patients before accepting in dialysis unit and ongoing screening of patients at regular interval to check for seroconversion, and having separate dialysis units with separate dialysis machines, dialyzer reuse systems, and dedicated staff for seropositive and seronegative patients. Blood transfusion should be done only when extremely necessary.

Hepatitis B Virus

Hepatitis B virus (HBV) is the most efficiently transmitted pathogen in the dialysis setting. HBV infection from an exposure occurs at a rate

Table 15.2 Prevalence of HBV in dialysis unit in India

Study by	Prevalence of HBV in dialysis unit (%)
Jaiswal et al. [31]	7.45
Sudan et al. [32]	6
Chandra et al. [33]	7
Chawla et al. [34]	5.41

of up to 30 %. Widespread implementation of recommendations for control of hepatitis B in hemodialysis setting has resulted in sharp decrease in the incidence and prevalence of HBV infection among dialysis patients [29].

Epidemiology

During the late 1970s, HBV infection was endemic in maintenance hemodialysis units and outbreaks were common. Subsequently, due to measures taken, the incidence and prevalence of HBV infection among maintenance hemodialysis patients in the United States has declined to 0.12 % and 1 %, respectively [30]. The prevalence of HBV in studies from India has also shown a reducing trend over time (Table 15.2). Newly acquired HBV infections were reported by 2.8 % of US hemodialysis centers, and 27.3 % of centers reported one or more patients with chronically infected patients [30]. According to the Indian CKD registry (as of December 2011), the prevalence of HBsAg-positive patients in hemodialysis patients is 3 %.

The chronically infected patient is central to the epidemiology of HBV transmission. HBV is transmitted by exposure of either skin or mucosa to infectious blood or body fluids that contain blood. All hepatitis B surface antigen (HBsAg)-positive persons who are also positive for hepatitis B e antigen (HBeAg) have a high level of HBV circulating in their blood. HBV is relatively stable in the environment and has been shown to remain viable for at least a week on environmental surfaces at room temperature [35–37]. So, blood-contaminated surfaces that are not routinely cleaned and disinfected (like dialysis machine control panel and doorknobs) represent a reservoir for HBV transmission [38]. Dialysis staff members can cause transfer of virus to susceptible

patients from surfaces in the absence of visible blood and still cause infection [35, 36, 38].

Most HBV outbreaks among hemodialysis patients occur due to cross-contamination of patients by use of multiple-dose vials for multiple patients and by utilizing same staff handling both HBV-positive and HBV-negative patients simultaneously [39, 40].

Despite the low incidence of HBV infection among hemodialysis patients, constant vigilance is essential to prevent HBV outbreaks to occur in maintenance hemodialysis centers. It is imperative that all the CKD patients when first seen should be vaccinated against HBV. Most of the time, outbreaks happen due to either failure to routinely screen patients for HBsAg or routinely review results of testing to identify infected patients, assignment of staff members to the simultaneous care of both infected and susceptible patients, or due to sharing of drug supplies, especially multidose medication vials, among patients.

Other risk factors for acquiring HBV infection include injection drug use, sexual and household exposure to HBV-infected contacts, exposure to multiple sexual partners, male homosexual activity, and perinatal exposure. These should be explained to dialysis patients in detail. Those dialysis patients who have active HBV infection (HBsAg positive) should be informed that their sexual partners and household contacts should be vaccinated [41, 42].

Screening and Diagnostic Tests

Tests related to HBV infection include HB$_S$Ag and antibody to HBsAg (anti-HBs), antibody to HBcAg (anti-HBc), and hepatitis B early antigen (HBeAg) and antibody to HBeAg (anti-HBe). HBV infection can also be detected, using qualitative or quantitative tests for HBV DNA, primarily used for HBV-infected patients being managed with antiviral therapy (Table 15.3).

In individuals who recover from HBV infection, HBsAg disappears from the blood, and anti-HBs antibodies develop during convalescence, usually within 4–6 months. The persistence of anti-HBs indicates immunity from HBV infection. If a person has recovered from natural

Table 15.3 Serological test results for hepatitis B virus infection [43]

	Total	IgM	Anti-	
HBsAg	anti-HBc	anti-HBc	HBs	Interpretation
Serological markers				
−	−	−	−	Susceptible, never infected
+	−	−	−	Acute ongoing infection, early incubation
+	+	+	−	Acute infection
−	+	+	−	Acute resolving infection
−	+	−	+	Past infection, recovered and immune
+	+	−	−	Chronic infection
−	+	−	−	False positive (i.e., susceptible), past infection, or low-level chronic
−	−	−	+	Immune if titer ≥10 mIU/ml

infection, he/she will be positive for both anti-HBc and anti-HBs, whereas only anti-HBs will be present in patients who are successfully vaccinated against hepatitis B.

Individuals who do not recover from HBV infection and become chronically infected remain HBsAg positive (and anti-HBc positive), although up to 2 % might eventually clear HBsAg and might usually develop anti-HBs [42, 44].

Another antigen, HBeAg, can be detected in the serum of individuals with acute or chronic HBV infection. The presence of HBeAg correlates with viral replication and high levels of virus (i.e., high infectivity). Anti-HBe antibodies develop on loss of replicating virus and with lower levels of virus. However, all HBsAg-positive patients should be considered potentially infectious, regardless of their HBeAg or anti-HBe status.

Before admission to the hemodialysis unit, the HBV serological status (i.e., HBsAg, total anti-HBc, and anti-HBs) of all patients should be known. For patients transferred from another unit, test results should be obtained before the patient transfer. If a patient's HBV serological status is not known at the time of admission, testing should be completed within 7 days.

To prevent HBV transmission among hemodialysis patients, certain recommendations were made which included [45] the following:

1. General precautions for staff and patients:
   (a) Serological screening of patients (and staff members) for HBV infection, including monthly testing of all susceptible patients for HBsAg.
   (b) Anti-HBSAb levels should be tested yearly in all immunized patients.
   (c) Isolation of HB$_s$Ag-positive patients.
   (d) Assignment of staff members to HBsAg-positive patients and not to HBV-susceptible patients during the same shift.
   (e) Assignment of dialysis equipment to HBsAg-positive patients that is not shared with HBV-susceptible patients.
   (f) Assignment of a supply tray to each patient (regardless of serological status).
   (g) Cleansing of dialysis machines and blood/body fluid contaminated areas with 1 % sodium hypochlorite (bleach) solution.
   (h) Dialyzer reuse prohibited for HBV-positive patients.
2. Universal precautions:
   (a) Staff must wear fluid-impermeable garments.
   (b) Gloves are to be used whenever there is potential for exposure to blood or body fluids.
   (c) Gloves must be changed and hands washed between patients.
   (d) Protective eyewear and face shields are worn when there is potential for splashing of blood (e.g., initiation and discontinuation of dialysis, changing the blood circuit).
   (e) No recapping of contaminated needles; prompt disposal in appropriate container.
   (f) No eating or drinking in dialysis unit.
3. Exposure to blood:
   (a) Testing for HB$_s$Ag and HB$_s$Ab at time of incident and 6 weeks later.
   (b) If HB$_s$Ag status of source patient is positive or unknown, administer hepatitis B immune globulin.

Hepatitis B Vaccination

All patients susceptible to HBV infection must be vaccinated. Anti-HBs should be tested 1–2 months after last dose of HBV vaccine to check for adequate titers of antibodies: if anti-HBs >10 mIU/ml, the patient should be considered immune and be tested annually. If anti-HBs <10 mIU/ml, the patient should be given three additional doses of HBV vaccine and re-tested for anti-HBs antibody titers. If the anti-HBs antibody level in an immune patient reduces below 10 mIU/ml, booster dose of the vaccine should be given and annual testing should continue. CKD patients are known to be poor seroconverters and may require a minimum of five doses for primary vaccination.

Management of Hepatitis B-Infected Patients

It is essential that HBsAg-positive patients should undergo hemodialysis in a separate room designated for HBsAg-positive patients only. They should use dedicated machines, equipment, and supplies, and most importantly staff members should not care for both HBsAg-positive and susceptible patients at the same time (shift) or while the HBsAg-positive patient is in the treatment area. Dialyzers should not be reused on HBsAg-positive patients because HBV is efficiently transmitted through occupational exposure to blood and reprocessing dialyzers from HBsAg-positive patients might place HBV-susceptible staff members at increased risk for infection.

HBV chronically infected patients (i.e., those who are HBsAg positive, total anti-HBc positive, and IgM anti-HBc negative) are infectious to others and are at risk for chronic liver disease. They should be counseled on how to prevent transmission to others, especially for those who are their household and sexual partners. Household contacts and sexual partners should be advised to receive hepatitis B vaccine. The HBsAg-positive patient should also be evaluated for the presence or development of chronic liver disease. It is recommended that individuals with chronic liver disease be vaccinated against the hepatitis A virus (HAV), if susceptible, to

Table 15.4 Prevalence of HCV in India

Study by	Prevalence of HCV in dialysis unit (%)
Salunkhe et al. [49]	45
Chadha et al. [50]	12.1
Sumathi et al. [51]	37.5
Agarwal et al. [52]	42
Jaiswal et al. [31]	30
Reddy et al. [53]	9.93

prevent any additional injury to the liver. HBV chronically infected patients do not require any routine follow-up testing for purposes of infection control. However, annual testing for HBsAg is reasonable to detect the small percentage of HBV-infected patients who might lose their HBsAg.

Hepatitis C Virus

Hepatitis C virus (HCV) is a single-stranded RNA virus belonging to the family Flaviviridae [46]. It is another efficiently transmitted blood-borne viral pathogen in the dialysis setting although not as efficiently transmitted as HBV. HCV infection from an exposure occurs at a rate of up to 1 %. The recommended infection control practices do prevent transmission among hemodialysis patients [45, 47, 48]. However, both outbreaks and new acquisition of HCV infection continue to occur among maintenance hemodialysis patients.

Epidemiology

Data are limited on the current incidence and prevalence of HCV infection among maintenance hemodialysis patients. It is the most common hepatotropic viral infection in patients on hemodialysis. The prevalence of HCV in studies from India has shown a decreasing trend over time (Table 15.4). Incidence of newly acquired HCV infections is 0.34 % in United States while the prevalence of anti-HCV-positive patients is 7.8 % [30]. According to the Indian CKD registry (as of December 2011), the prevalence of anti-HCV-positive patients in dialysis patients is 2.8 %.

HCV is moderately stable in the environment and can survive drying and environmental exposure to room temperature for at least 16 h [54]. HCV is most efficiently transmitted by direct percutaneous exposure to blood, and like HBV, the chronically infected patient is central to the epidemiology of HCV transmission. Risk factors associated with HCV infection among hemodialysis patients include blood transfusions from unscreened donors, intravenous drug abuse, low staff to patient ratios, and number of years on dialysis [55, 56].

The number of years on dialysis is the major risk factor that is independently associated with higher rates of HCV infection. As the duration spent by patients on dialysis increased, their prevalence of HCV infection increased from an average of 12 % for patients receiving dialysis <5 years to an average of 37 % for patients receiving dialysis >5 years [55, 57]. The studies and investigations of dialysis-associated outbreaks of HCV infection indicate that HCV transmission most likely occurs because of inadequate infection control practices [58]. Other reported risk factors for acquiring HCV include injection drug use, receipt of unscreened blood via transfusion, exposure to an HCV-infected sexual partner or household contact, multiple sexual partners, and perinatal exposure [59, 60]. The efficiency of transmission in settings involving sexual or household exposure to infected contacts is low, and the magnitude of risk and the circumstances under which these exposures result in transmission are not well defined.

Screening and Diagnostic Tests

Anti-HCV screening tests include three immunoassays: two enzyme immunoassays (EIA) and one enhanced chemiluminescence immunoassay (CIA). Although no true confirmatory test has been developed, supplemental tests for specificity are available which include a serological anti-HCV assay, the strip immunoblot assay (Chiron RIBAW HCV 3.0 SIA, Chiron Corp., Emeryville, California), and nucleic acid tests (NAT) for HCV RNA (including reverse transcriptase polymerase chain reaction [RT-PCR] amplification and transcription-mediated amplification [TMA]).

Anti-HCV testing includes initial screening with an EIA immunoassay. However, interpretation of the results of EIAs that screen for anti-HCV is limited by several factors: (1) these assays will not detect anti-HCV in approximately 10 % of persons infected with HCV; (2) these assays do not distinguish between acute, chronic, and past infection; (3) in the acute phase of hepatitis C, there may be a prolonged interval between onset of illness and seroconversion; and (4) in populations with a low prevalence of infection, the rate of false positivity for anti-HCV is high. If the screening test is positive, either a high screening test-positive signal-to-cut-off ratio or supplemental testing with a test with high specificity should be performed to verify the results. Among hemodialysis patients, the proportion of false-positive screening test results averages approximately 15 %. For this reason, one should not rely exclusively on a positive anti-HCV screening test to determine whether a person has been infected with HCV.

Routine testing of hemodialysis patients for anti-HCV on admission and every 6 months has been recommended [61]. For routine HCV testing of hemodialysis patients, the anti-HCV screening immunoassay is recommended, and if positive, supplemental anti-HCV testing using RIBA or NAT should be done. RIBA is recommended rather than NAT because the serological assay can be performed on the same serum or plasma sample collected for the screening anti-HCV screening assay.

In addition, in certain situations the HCV RNA results can be negative in persons with active infection. As the titer of anti-HCV increases during acute infection, the titer of HCV RNA declines [62]. Thus HCV RNA is not detectable in certain persons during the acute phase of their infection, but this finding can be transient and chronic infection can develop [63]. In addition, intermittent HCV positivity has been observed among patients with chronic HCV infection [64]. Therefore, the significance of a single negative HCV RNA result is unknown, and the need for further investigation or follow-up is determined by verifying anti-HCV status (Table 15.5).

Table 15.5 Interpretation of test results for HCV infection [65]

Anti-HCV positive
Anti-HCV screening test positive with a high signal-to-cut off ratio
Anti-HCV screening test positive with RIBA positive or NAT positive
Anti-HCV screening test positive, NAT negative, RIBA positive
Indicates past or current HCV infection
Indicates current (active) infection, but significance of single HCV RNA negative result is unknown; it does not differentiate intermittent viremia from resolved infection
All anti-HCV-positive persons should receive counseling and undergo medical evaluation, including additional testing for the presence of virus and liver disease
Anti-HCV testing generally does not need to be repeated once a positive anti-HCV result has been confirmed
Anti-HCV negative
Anti-HCV screening test negative
Anti-HCV screening test positive, RIBA negative
Anti-HCV screening test positive, NAT negative, RIBA negative
Individual is considered uninfected
No further evaluation or follow-up for HCV is required unless recent infection is suspected or other evidence exists to indicate HCV infection (e.g., abnormal liver enzyme levels in immunocompromised persons or persons with other etiology for their liver disease)
Anti-HCV indeterminate
Anti-HCV screening test positive, RIBA indeterminate
Anti-HCV screening test positive, NAT negative, RIBA indeterminate
Indicates that the HCV antibody status cannot be determined
Can indicate a false-positive anti-HCV screening test result, the most likely interpretation in those at low risk for HCV infection; such persons are HCV RNA negative
Can occur as a transient finding in recently infected individuals who are in the process of seroconversion; such individuals usually are HCV RNA positive
Can be a persistent finding in an individual chronically infected with HCV; such persons are usually HCV RNA positive
If NAT is not performed, another sample should be collected for repeat anti-HCV testing (≥ 1 month later)

If ALT levels are persistently abnormal in anti-HCV-negative patients in the absence of another etiology, testing for HCV RNA should be considered. Blood samples collected for NAT should not contain heparin, which interferes with the accurate performance of this assay.

To prevent HCV transmission among hemodialysis patients, recommendations for prevention of HBV infections in addition to the following should be followed [45]:

1. Serological screening of patients (and staff members) should include monthly ALT and 6-month anti-HCV for all anti-HCV-negative patients.
2. Isolation is not necessary for HCV-infected patients
3. Dialyzer reuse can be done in anti-HCV-positive patients.

Management of HCV-Infected Dialysis Patients

The purpose of routine testing is to monitor potential transmission within centers and ensure that appropriate practices are being properly and consistently used. HCV-positive patients need not be isolated from other patients or dialyzed separately on dedicated machines. Unlike HBV, HCV is not transmitted efficiently through occupational exposures. Thus, reprocessing dialyzers from HCV-positive patients should not place staff members at increased risk for infection [66, 67]. HCV-positive patients should be evaluated for presence or development of chronic liver disease. They should be told about ways to prevent further transmission of infection to others. If they have chronic liver disease, they should be vaccinated for hepatitis A.

Hepatitis Delta Virus

Hepatitis delta virus (HDV) is a relatively small defective virus that causes infection in persons with active HBV infection only. The prevalence of HDV infection is low in the United States, with rates <1 % among HBsAg-positive persons in the general population and >10 % among HBsAg-positive persons with repeated exposures (e.g., injecting drug users, persons with hemophilia) [68]. Data from India regarding incidence and prevalence of HDV infection among hemodialysis patients is lacking.

HDV infection may occur as either coinfection with HBV or as a super infection in a person with chronic HBV infection. Coinfections usually resolve, but super infections frequently result in chronic HDV infection and severe disease. High mortality rates are associated with both types of infection. Because HDV depends on an HBV-infected host for replication, prevention of HBV infection will prevent HDV infection in a person susceptible to HBV. Patients known to be infected with HDV should be isolated from all other dialysis patients, especially those who are HBsAg positive.

Human Immunodeficiency Virus Infection

The proportion of patients with known human immunodeficiency virus (HIV) infection among dialysis patients is around 1.5 % in the United States [30]. HIV is transmitted by blood and other body fluids that contain blood. No patient-to-patient transmission of HIV has been reported in a US hemodialysis center. Data from India is lacking in this aspect. However, there have been reports of transmission of HIV among patients in other countries. All of these outbreaks have been attributed to several breaks in infection control: (1) reuse of access needles and inadequately disinfected equipment, (2) sharing of syringes among patients, and (3) sharing of dialyzers among different patients [69]. HIV infection is usually diagnosed with assays that measure antibody to HIV, and a repeatedly positive EIA

test should be confirmed by Western blot or other confirmatory test.

Management
Routine testing for HIV infection for purposes of infection control is not recommended in populations with low endemicity. Infection control precautions recommended for all hemodialysis patients are sufficient to prevent HIV transmission between patients. HIV-infected patients do not have to be isolated from other patients or dialyzed separately on dedicated machines. In addition, they can participate in dialyzer reuse programs, because HIV is not transmitted efficiently through occupational exposures. Reprocessing dialyzers from HIV-positive patients should not place staff members at increased risk for infection.

Other Infections

These include other bacterial infections, pneumonia, UTI, intra-abdominal infections, fungal infections, and tuberculosis.

1. *Pneumonia:* It is a common cause of hospitalization in ESRD patients, seen more commonly in elderly (>65 year age) and those who are malnourished. This is common in view of transient hypoxemia occurring during dialysis procedure (due to margination of leukocytes in the pulmonary vasculature and carbon dioxide losses) and also because of the institutional setting (due to exposure to other patients).

    Pneumonia in dialysis patient carries a poor prognosis and is often the antecedent to cardiovascular death. Mortality rate for pneumonia in dialysis patients is 14–16 times higher than in general population. Risk factors for pneumonia in dialysis patients include chronic obstructive pulmonary disease, inability to transfer or ambulate, hemodialysis as initial therapy, advanced age ($\geq$75 years), low serum albumin, and body mass index <18.5 kg.m^2 or $\geq$30 kg/m^2 [70]. Influenza vaccination is recommended in patients on dialysis as it has been shown to be associated with statistically significant decrease in the risk of death and hospitalization.

2. *Urinary Tract Infection (UTI):* In dialysis patients the incidence of UTI is high, especially in patients with polycystic kidney disease. In patients with a neurogenic bladder (e.g., diabetic patients), pyocystis (pus in the defunctionalized bladder) may be an unsuspected source of infection.

3. *Intra-abdominal Infections:* Diverticulosis and diverticulitis occur commonly in dialysis patients and especially in those with polycystic kidney disease. Strangulated hernia is also frequently encountered. Intestinal infarction can occur as a complication of hypotension occurring during a dialysis session or between dialyses; bowel infarction should always be suspected in a dialysis patient with unexplained, refractory septic shock.

4. *Tuberculosis:* The incidence of tuberculosis has been estimated to be as much as tenfold higher among hemodialysis patients than among the general population. Tuberculosis in hemodialysis patients is frequently extrapulmonary; disseminated disease may occur in the absence of chest x-ray abnormalities. Delayed skin hypersensitivity to tuberculin reagent is often absent or diminished due to cutaneous anergy making it difficult to diagnose.

   CDC recommends that all patients on dialysis should be screened for tuberculosis at baseline and whenever exposure is suspected. When the index of suspicion for tuberculosis is high, presumptive therapy with antitubercular agents is sometimes warranted. Mortality in dialysis patients with tuberculosis has been reported to be as high as 40 %.

5. *Other Bacterial/Fungal Infections:* Contact transmission of bacterial/fungal infections can be prevented by hand hygiene, glove use, and disinfection of environmental surfaces [71]. Infection control precautions recommended for all hemodialysis patients are adequate to prevent transmission for most patients infected or colonized with pathogenic bacteria, including antimicrobial-resistant strains.

   However, additional precautions should be considered for treatment of patients who might be at increased risk for transmitting pathogenic bacteria. Such patients include those with either an infected skin wound with drainage that is not contained by dressings (the drainage does not have to be culture positive for MRSA or VRE or any specific pathogen) or fecal incontinence or diarrhea uncontrolled with personal hygiene measures. For these patients, staff members treating the patient should wear a separate gown over their usual clothing and remove the gown when finished caring for the patient and dialyze the patient at a station away from the main flow of traffic and with as few adjacent stations as possible (e.g., at the end or corner of the unit).

Vancomycin is used commonly in dialysis patients, in part because vancomycin can be conveniently administered to patients when they come in for hemodialysis treatments. Vancomycin is not indicated for therapy (chosen for dosing convenience) of infections because of β-lactam-sensitive gram-positive microorganisms in patients with renal failure. Depending on the situation, alternative antimicrobials (e.g., cephalosporins) with dosing intervals greater than 48 h, which would allow post-dialytic dosing, could be used. Recent studies suggest that cefazolin given three times a week in the dialysis unit provides adequate blood levels and could be used to treat many infections in hemodialysis patients [72].

Conclusions

Hemodialysis patients have unique vulnerability to healthcare-associated infections. This is because of a number of human, environmental, and procedural factors related to the hemodialysis setting, in addition to a multitude of patient comorbidities. Establishing an infection prevention and control program which includes a bundle of strategies and interventions that are consistently performed will reduce the risk for both employees and patients. These include environmental cleaning/disinfection, equipment cleaning/disinfection, hand hygiene, immunizations and screening for patients and employees, medication/injection safety, patient/family/employee education, pre-/postsurgical infection prevention, standard/transmission-based precautions, vascular access, infection prevention during insertion and care, water treatment/testing, and infection surveillance.

Standard empiric protocols for the treatment of infection in dialysis settings should be replaced by a regime tailored to the local circumstances, the individual organism, and its antibiotic resistance pattern.

The prevalence of hepatitis C remains significantly higher in patients on hemodialysis and increased duration of dialysis therapy is associated with increased risk of seroconversion.

Inadequate antibody titers after vaccination against hepatitis B virus are a consistent and strong predictor of hepatitis B seroconversion.

Patients undergoing hemodialysis seem to be more susceptible to infections, such as pneumonia; vaccination against influenza mitigates the increased mortality in patients on hemodialysis.

References

1. Rajapurkar MM, John GT, Kirpalani AL, Abraham G, Agarwal SK, Almeida AF, et al. What do we know about chronic kidney disease in India: first report of the Indian CKD registry. BMC Nephrol. 2012;13:10.
2. Khan IH, Catto GR. Long-term complications of dialysis: infection. Kidney Int. 1993;41(Suppl):S143–8.
3. Favero MS, Petersen NJ, Carson LA, Bond WW, Hindman SH. Gram-negative water bacteria in hemodialysis systems. Health Lab Sci. 1975;12(4):321–34.
4. Basok A, Vorobiov M, Rogachev B, Avnon L, Toybin D, Hausmann M, et al. Spectrum of mycobacterial infections: tuberculosis and *Mycobacterium* other than tuberculosis in dialysis patients. Isr Med Assoc J. 2007;9(6):448–51.
5. Favero MS, Petersen NJ, Boyer KM, Carson LA, Bond WW. Microbial contamination of renal dialysis systems and associated health risks. Trans Am Soc Artif Intern Organs. 1974;20A:175–83.
6. Nystrand R. Microbiology of water and fluids for hemodialysis. J Chin Med Assoc. 2008;71(5):223–9.
7. Leitlinie für angewandte hygiene in dialysezentren. 2 Auflage. Arbeitskreis für angewandte hygiene in dialysezentren. Pabst Verlag. 2005. ISBN 3-89967-272-0. [In German].
8. Kawanishi H, Akiba T, Masakane I, Tomo T, Mineshima M, Kawasaki T, et al. Standard on microbiological management of fluids for hemodialysis and related therapies by the Japanese society for dialysis therapy 2008. Ther Apher Dial. 2009;13(2):161–6.
9. Svensk Läkemedelsstandard SLS 2007. Svenska farmakopékommittén, Uppsala. 2007. ISBN 91-973998-6-8. [In Swedish].
10. Canadian Standards Association. Water treatment equipment and water quality requirements for hemodialysis, CSA standard, vol. Z364.2.2-03. Mississauga: Canadian Standards Association; 2003.
11. AAMI. American national standard: reuse of hemodialyzers, ANSI/AAMI RD-47. Arlington: Association for the Advancement for Medical Instrumentation; 2008.
12. Arduino MJ. Microbiologic quality of water used for hemodialysis. Contemp Dial Nephrol. 1996;17:17–9.
13. Petersen NJ, Boyer KM, Carson LA, Favero MS. Pyrogenic reactions from inadequate disinfection of a dialysis fluid distribution system. Dialysis Transplant. 1978;7:52–7.
14. Bland LA, Favero MS, editors. Microbial contamination control strategies for hemodialysis systems, Plant, technology, and safety management, vol. 3. Oakbrook Terrace: Joint Commission on Accreditation of Healthcare Organizations; 1989.
15. Townsend TR, Wee SB, Bartlett J. Disinfection of hemodialysis machines. Dial Transplant. 1985;14:274–87.
16. Favero MS, Petersen NJ. Microbiologic guidelines for hemodialysis systems. Dial Transplant. 1977;6:34–6.
17. Alter MJ, Favero MS, Moyer LA, Bland LA. National surveillance of dialysis-associated diseases in the United States, 1989. ASAIO Trans. 1991;37(2):97–109.
18. Kaplowitz LG, Comstock JA, Landwehr DM, Dalton HP, Mayhall CG. A prospective study of infections in hemodialysis patients: patient hygiene and other risk factors for infection. Infect Control Hosp Epidemiol. 1988;9(12):534–41.
19. Tokars JI, Miller ER, Stein G. New national surveillance system for hemodialysis-associated infections: initial results. Am J Infect Control. 2002;30(5):288–95.
20. Klevens RM, Edwards JR, Andrus ML, Peterson KD, Dudeck MA, Horan TC. Dialysis surveillance report: National Healthcare Safety Network (NHSN)-data summary for 2006. Semin Dial. 2008;1(1):24–8.
21. Klevens RM, Tokars JI, Andrus M. Electronic reporting of infections associated with hemodialysis. Nephrol News Issues. 2005;19(7):37–843.
22. Bonomo RA, Rice D, Whalen C, Linn D, Eckstein E, Shlaes DM. Risk factors associated with permanent access-site infections in chronic hemodialysis patients. Infect Control Hosp Epidemiol. 1997;18(11):757–61.
23. NKF: III. NKF-K/DOQI clinical practice guidelines for vascular access: update 2000. Am J Kidney Dis. 2001;37(1 Suppl 1):S137–81.
24. NKF. Clinical practice guidelines for vascular access. Am J Kidney Dis. 2006;48 Suppl 1:S248–73.
25. CDC. Guidelines for the prevention of intravascular catheter-related infections. MMWR. 2002;51(RR-10):1–29.
26. Dinwiddie L. Cleansing agents used for hemodialysis catheter care. Nephrol Nurs J. 2002;29(6):599–613.
27. Mermel LA. Prevention of intravascular catheter infections – insights and prospects for hemodialysis catheters. Nephrologie. 2001;22(8):449–51.
28. Mermel LA, Farr BM, Sherertz RJ, Raad II, O'Grady N, Harris JS, et al. Guidelines for the management of

intravascular catheter-related infections. Clin Infect Dis. 2001;32(9):1249–72.

29. Alter MJ, Favero MS, Maynard JE. Impact of infection control strategies on the incidence of dialysis-associated hepatitis in the United States. J Infect Dis. 1986;153(6):1149–51.

30. Finelli L, Miller JT, Tokars JI, Alter MJ, Arduino MJ. National surveillance of dialysis-associated diseases in the United States, 2002. Semin Dial. 2005;18(1):52–61.

31. Jaiswal S, Chitnis D, Salgia P, Sepaha A, Pandit C. Prevalence of the hepatitis virus among chronic renal failure patients on hemodialysis in central India. Dial Transplant. 2002;31:234–8.

32. Sudan SS, Sharma RK. Prevalence of hepatitis B & C in CRF patients on haemodialysis. http://www.bhj.org.in/journal/2003_4502_april/prevalence_301.htm. Accessed 15 Dec 2012.

33. Chandra M, Khaja MN, Hussain MM, Poduri CD, Farees N, Habeeb MA, et al. Prevalence of hepatitis B and hepatitis C viral infections in Indian patients with chronic renal failure. Intervirology. 2004;47:374–6.

34. Chawla NS, Sajiv CT, Pawar G, Pawar B. Hepatitis B and C Virus infections associated with renal replacement therapy in patients with end stage renal disease in a tertiary care hospital in India – prevalence, risk factors and outcome. Indian J Nephrol. 2005;15:205–13.

35. Alter HJ, Seeff LB, Kaplan PM, McAuliffe VJ, Wright EC, Gerin JL, et al. Type B hepatitis: the infectivity of blood positive for e antigen and DNA polymerase after accidental needlestick exposure. N Engl J Med. 1976;295(17):909–13.

36. Bond WW, Favero MS, Petersen NJ, Gravelle CR, Ebert JW, Maynard JE. Survival of hepatitis B virus after drying and storage for one week. Lancet. 1981;1(8219):550–1.

37. Favero MS, Bond WW, Petersen NJ, Berquist KR, Maynard JE. Detection methods for study of the stability of hepatitis B antigen on surfaces. J Infect Dis. 1974;129(2):210–12.

38. Favero MS, Maynard JE, Petersen NJ, Boyer KM, Bond WW, Berquist KR, et al. Letter: hepatitis-B antigen on environmental surfaces. Lancet. 1973;2(7843):1455.

39. Alter MJ, Ahtone J, Maynard JE. Hepatitis B virus transmission associated with a multiple-dose vial in a hemodialysis unit. Ann Int Med. 1983;99(3):330–3.

40. Carl M, Francis DP, Maynard JE. A common-source outbreak of hepatitis B in a hemodialysis unit. Dial Transplant. 1983;12:222–9.

41. Rangel MC, Coronado VG, Euler GL, Strikas RA. Vaccine recommendations for patients on chronic dialysis. The Advisory Committee on Immunization Practices and the American Academy of Pediatrics. Semin Dial. 2000;13(2):101–7.

42. Mast EE, Weinbaum CM, Fiore AE, Alter MJ, Bell BP, Finelli L, et al. A comprehensive immunization strategy to eliminate transmission of hepatitis B virus infection in the United States: recommendations of the Advisory Committee on Immunization Practices (ACIP) Part II: immunization of adults. MMWR. 2006;55(RR-16):1–33. quiz CE31–34.

43. Hoofnagle JH, Di Bisceglie AM. Serologic diagnosis of acute and chronic hepatitis. Sem Liver Dis. 1991;11(2):73–83.

44. McMahon BJ, Alberts SR, Wainwright RB, Bulkow L, Lanier AP. Hepatitis B-related sequelae. Prospective study in 1400 hepatitis B surface antigen-positive Alaska native carriers. Arch Int Med. 1990;150(5):1051–4.

45. CDC. Recommendations for preventing transmission of infections among chronic hemodialysis patients. MMWR. 2001;50(RR-5):1–43.

46. Bendinelli M, Pistello M, Maggi F, Vatteroni M. Blood-borne hepatitis viruses: hepatitis B, C, D, and G viruses and TT virus. In: Specter S, Hodinka RL, Young SA, editors. Clinical virology manual. 3rd ed. Washington, DC: ASM Press; 2000.

47. CDC. Recommendations for prevention and control of hepatitis C virus (HCV) infection and HCV-related chronic disease. MMWR. 1998;47(RR19):1–39.

48. Moyer LA, Alter MJ. Hepatitis C virus in the hemodialysis setting: a review with recommendations for control. Semin Dial. 1994;7:124–7.

49. Salunkhe PN, Naik SR, Semwal SN, Naik S, Kher V. Prevalence of antibodies to hepatitis C virus in HBsAg negative haemodialysis patients. Indian J Gastroenterol. 1992;11(4):164–5.

50. Chadha MS, Arankalle VA, Jha J, Banerjee K. Prevalence of hepatitis B and C virus infection among hemodialysis in Pune (Western India). Vox Sang. 1993;64:127–8.

51. Sumathi S, Valliammai T, Thyagarajan SP, Malathy S, Madanagopalan N, Sankarnarayan V, et al. Prevalence of hepatitis C virus infection in liver diseases, renal diseases and voluntary blood donors in South India. Indian J Med Microbial. 1993;11(4):291–7.

52. Agarwal SK, Dash SC, Irshad MC. Hepatitis C virus infection during hemodialysis in India. J Assoc Phys India. 1999;47:1139–43.

53. Reddy AK, Murthy KV, Lakshmi V. Prevalence of HCV infection in patients on haemodialysis: survey by antibody and core antigen detection. Indian J Med Microbiol. 2005;23:106–10.

54. Kamili S, Krawczynski K, McCaustland K, Li X, Alter MJ. Infectivity of hepatitis C virus in plasma after drying and storing at room temperature. Infect Control Hosp Epidemiol. 2007;28(5):519–24.

55. Niu MT, Coleman PJ, Alter MJ. Multicenter study of hepatitis C virus infection in chronic hemodialysis patients and hemodialysis center staff members. Am J Kidney Dis. 1993;22(4):568–73.

56. Petrosillo N, Gilli P, Serraino D, Dentico P, Mele A, Ragni P, et al. Prevalence of infected patients and under-staffing have a role in hepatitis C virus transmission in dialysis. Am J Kidney Dis. 2001;37(5):1004–10.

57. Selgas R, Martinez-Zapico R, Bajo MA, Romero JR, Munoz J, Rion C, et al. Prevalence of hepatitis

C antibodies (HCV) in a dialysis population at one center. Perit Dial Int. 1992;12(1):28–30.

58. Thompson ND, Novack RT, Datta D, Cotter S, Arduino MJ, Patel PR, et al. Hepatitis C virus transmission in the hemodialysis setting: importance of infection control practices and aseptic technique. Infect Control Hosp Epidemiol. 2009;30:900–3.

59. Alter MJ. The epidemiology of acute and chronic hepatitis C. Clin Liver Dis. 1997;1:559–68.

60. Alter MJ. Prevention of spread of hepatitis C. Hepatology. 2002;26(5 Suppl 1):S93–8.

61. CDC. Guidelines for laboratory testing and result testing for hepatitis C virus. MMWR. 2003;52(RR3):1–15.

62. Busch MP, Kleinman SH, Jackson B, Stramer SL, Hewlett I, Preston S. Committee report. Nucleic acid amplification testing of blood donors for transfusion-transmitted infectious diseases: report of the Interorganizational Task Force on Nucleic Acid Amplification Testing of Blood Donors. Transfusion. 2000;40(2):143–59.

63. Williams IT, Gretch D, Fleenor M. Hepatitis C RNA concentration and chronic hepatitis in a cohort of patients followed after developing acute hepatitis C. In: Margolis HS, Alter MJ, Liang TJ, Dienstag JL, editors. Viral hepatitis and liver disease. Atlanta: International Medical Press; 2000. p. 341–4.

64. Thomas DL, Astemborski J, Rai RM, Anania FA, Schaeffer M, Galai N, et al. The natural history of hepatitis C virus infection: host, viral, and environmental factors. JAMA. 2000;284(4):450–6.

65. www.cdc.gov/hepatitis/HCV/PDFs/hcv_graph.pdf

66. Arduino MJ, Tokars JI, Lyerla R, et al. Preventing health-care associated transmission of bloodborne pathogens in hemodialysis facilities. Sem Infect Control. 2001;1(1):49–60.

67. Arduino MJ. How should dialyzers be reprocessed? Semin Dial. 1998;11(5):282–4.

68. Hadler SC, Fields HA. Hepatitis delta virus. In: Belshe BB, editor. Textbook of human virology. St. Louis: Mosby; 1991.

69. Favero MS. Transmission of HIV in dialysis units. ANNA J. 1993;20(5):599–600.

70. Guo H, Liu J, Collins AJ, Foley RN. Pneumonia in incident dialysis patients—the United States Renal Data System. Nephrol Dial Transplant. 2008;23(2):680–6.

71. CDC. Guideline for hand hygiene in health-care settings. MMWR. 2002;51 RR16

72. Fogel MA, Nussbaum PB, Feintzeig ID, Hunt WA, Gavin JP, Kim RC. Cefazolin in chronic hemodialysis patients: a safe, effective alternative to vancomycin. Am J Kidney Dis. 1998;32(3):401–9.

Monitoring of High-Risk Areas: Burn Units

16

Sarika Jain and Rajni Gaind

Introduction

Burns are one of the most common and devastating forms of trauma. Globally WHO estimates burn-related deaths to be 195,000 annually, and almost half occur in the Southeast Asia Region. In India, over 6–7 million people sustain moderate or severe burns per year. In 2008, over 410,000 burn injuries occurred in the United States of America, with approximately 40,000 requiring hospitalization [1]. Infection and sepsis are among the leading causes of mortality in burns, responsible for 75 % of all deaths [2]. Prevention and control of infections in burn patient is a challenge as several characteristics of burn patients (Table 16.1) make them particularly susceptible to infection; the environment in burn units (BUs) can become contaminated; and these organisms can be easily transmitted. Thus, BU can be a site of explosive and prolonged outbreaks caused by resistant organisms.

The guidelines issued by CDC do not address infection control specifically for the burn unit, and there is lack of consensus among BUs regarding infection control procedures and techniques necessary for burn patients.

S. Jain, M.D. • R. Gaind, M.D. (✉)
Department of Microbiology, VMMC and Safdarjung Hospital, New Delhi, India
e-mail: rgaind5@hotmail.com

Sources of Organisms

The reservoirs for agents causing infection are burn wound surfaces, endogenous normal gastrointestinal or upper respiratory tract flora of patients, or exogenous that is transferred from hospital environment or hands of health-care personnel (HCP) [3]. Burn wound is initially colonized with gram-positive organisms which are substituted with antibiotic susceptible gram-negative bacteria. With delay in closure of wound, infection with antibiotic-resistant bacteria or fungi sets in. Antimicrobial resistance contributes to increased morbidity, deaths, and health-care costs. Emergence of multiresistant organisms (MRO) of particular concern are methicillin-resistant *Staphylococcus aureus* (MRSA), vancomycin-resistant enterococcus (VRE), and gram-negative bacteria producing extended spectrum beta-lactamases, AmpC beta-lactamases, carbapenemases such as KPC and NDM-1, or other metallo-beta-lactamases. Risk factors identified in patients colonized with drug-resistant organisms include prior use of third-generation cephalosporins and antibiotics active against anaerobes, prolonged hospital stay, associated immunosuppression, or underlying disease.

Among fungi, candida colonization is primarily endogenous, whereas molds are ubiquitous in the environment. Organisms associated with infection in burn patients are shown in Table 16.2.

Table 16.1 Factors influencing development of infections in burn patients

1. Local factors	Effects
a. Destruction skin barrier	Microbial colonization and infection
b. Protein-rich avascular necrotic tissue (eschar)	Favorable niche for microbial colonization and proliferation
c. The avascularity of the eschar	Impaired migration of host immune cells restricts delivery of systemically administered antimicrobial agents to the area
d. Toxic substances released by eschar tissue	Impair local host immune responses
2. Immunological response to burn injury	
Depression of local and systemic host cellular and humoral immune responses	State of immunosuppression that predisposes burn patients to infectious complications
3. Use of invasive procedures and devices	Predispose to systemic infections
4. Extended hospital stay and exposure to hospital environment	Increased risk of acquiring infections with multidrug-resistant bacteria

Table 16.2 Changing patterns of etiology of burn wound infections

NNIS, CDC 1974–1978 ($n=1,984$)	NNIS, CDC 1980–1998 ($n=1,834$)
Staphylococcus aureus (22.9)	Staphylococcus aureus (23.0)
Pseudomonas aeruginosa (20.9)	Pseudomonas aeruginosa (19.3)
Pseudomonas species (7.2)	Enterococci (11.0)
Escherichia coli (6.7)	Enterobacter species (9.6)
Group D streptococci (5.0)	Escherichia coli (7.2)
Enterococci (4.2)	Coagulase-negative staphylococci (4.3)
Klebsiella pneumoniae (3.7)	Candida albicans (3.5)
Serratia marcescens (3.1)	Serratia marcescens (3.5)
Enterobacter cloacae (3.0)	Klebsiella pneumoniae (2.6)
Proteus mirabilis (2.8)	Others (16.0)
Enterobacter species (2.5)	
Klebsiella species (2.2)	
Staphylococcus epidermidis (1.4)	
Group A streptococci (1.1)	
Enterobacter aerogenes (1.0)	
Candida albicans (1.3)	

Adapted from Mayhall, CID 2003 [3]
Note: Figures in parenthesis indicate percentage
NNIS National Nosocomial Infections Study, *CDC* Center for Disease Control

Mode of Nosocomial Pathogen Transmission

In burn patients, transmission takes place by hands of HCP or from contact with inadequately decontaminated equipment. Burn patients with open wounds are prone to colonization from organisms in the environment as well as in their propensity to disperse organisms into the surrounding environment. In almost all cases, the colonized patients are thought to be a major reservoir for the epidemic strains.

Reservoir of nosocomial pathogens include hydrotherapy units and common treatment areas, where water used is contaminated with gram-negative organisms either intrinsically and/or by organisms from other patients. This aquatic environment is difficult to decontaminate due to continuous reinoculation from patient's wound flora and tendency to form a protective glycocalyx in water pipes and drains, making them resistant to action of disinfectants [4]. Adequate cleaning of patient care equipments and common treatment area is difficult to achieve between patients on daily basis, and monitoring techniques are often insufficient to provide timely detection of contamination. Patients own flora (colonized wound) may spread via water or hands of HCP to colonize other critical sites (central venous catheter). Hands and personnel protective equipment like gowns of the HCP become contaminated as the surfaces are often heavily contaminated with organism from the patient, and same may be transmitted if strict barriers are not maintained. In case of outbreaks, several factors contribute to dissemination of pathogens.

Epidemiology of Infections in Burn Patients

The changing epidemiology of infection in critically ill, severely burned patient is a result of greater understanding of pathophysiology of infections and improved techniques of wound management. The use of topical antimicrobials controls the microbial density in burn wound, thereby decreasing the occurrence of burn wound infection and also permitting burn wound excision to be carried out, with marked reduction in intraoperative bacteremia and endotoxemia. These procedures have decreased the incidence of invasive burn wound sepsis as the cause of death in patients at BUs (BU) from 60 % in the 1960s to only 6 % in the 1980s [5].

The most important factors that influence morbidity and mortality from burn wound infection and sepsis include the following:
- Large TSBA wound
- Significant amounts of full-thickness burns
- Prolonged open wounds and delayed initial burn wound care
- Duration of hospitalization
- Use of invasive devices

Patients with total body surface area (TBSA) burn injuries $\geq$30 % had greater incidence of bacteremia, UTI, pneumonia, and invasive burn

wound infection as compared to those with <30 % TBSA [6]. Invasive diagnostic and therapeutic procedures predispose burn patient to hospital-acquired infections. In a prospective study in a BU of a tertiary care center in North India, the infection density was 36.2 infections per 1,000 patient days [2]. Catheter-associated bloodstream infection (CLABSI) occurs with far greater frequency in burn patients than in other patient groups. Catheters are prone to colonization with hematogenous seeding of organisms from contaminated burn wound or due to close presence of central lines near burned wounds. Long-term central lines are also susceptible to biofilm formation and are difficult to eradicate by antimicrobial therapy, necessitating removal of these precious catheters. Frequent manipulation or breach in aseptic techniques while placement of line or in handling of these catheters also leads to colonization of these catheters. Data submitted from burn intensive care units to the National Nosocomial Infections Surveillance (NNIS) system at the CDC during 2006–2008 showed the highest rate of CLABSI in BU (pooled mean of 5.3) compared to all other critical care units (ranging from 1.2 to 2.6). Similarly, VAP rates were much higher in burn patients than any other unit (pooled mean 7.4 vs. 0.6 to 6.5) [7]. The frequency of infection in burn patient is shown in Figs. 16.1 and 16.2.

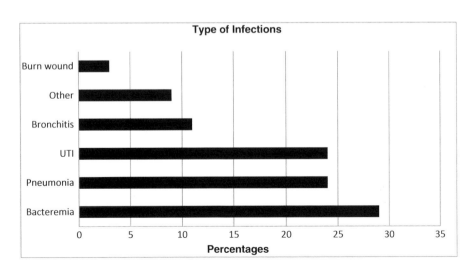

Fig. 16.1 Frequency of various infections in burn patients. Note: The frequency of infection by site expressed as a percentage of all infections complicating thermal injury (Adapted from United States Army Institute of Surgical Research, 1991–1995) [12]

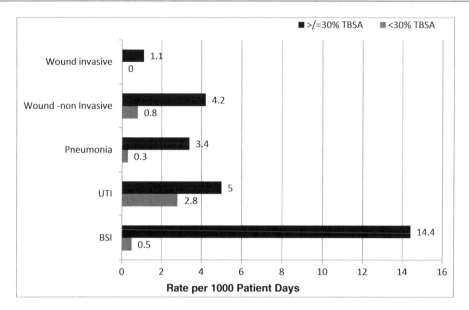

Fig. 16.2 Frequency of infections by site according to total body surface area (TBSA) burn. Incidence of infection by site at Shriners Hospitals for Children, Boston, from January 1996 to December 2000 [6]. Rates are infections per 1,000 patient days. *BSI* bloodstream infection, *UTI* urinary tract infection, *TBSA* total body surface area burn

Culture and Surveillance Studies

Burn wound flora and antibiotic susceptibilities change during the course of hospitalization, and hence, it is imperative to perform routine surveillance cultures of burn wound infections periodically for the following:

1. Early identification of organisms colonizing the wound
2. Monitoring the effectiveness of current management
3. Guiding perioperative or empirical antibiotic therapy
4. Early detection of cross-colonization to prevent transmission

These should be obtained on admission as a baseline data, then 2–3 times in a week until the burn wound has been excised, and thereafter once weekly to monitor change in microbial flora.

Surveillance cultures, e.g., nasal and groin swab for MRSA and fecal carriage for VRE, ESBL, and carbapenemase-producing Enterobacteriaceae, may be useful for identification of antibiotic-resistant strain for implementation of control measures. Surveillance of hospital-associated infection and its feedback to clinicians has been shown to reduce nosocomial infection rates. Systematic and timely collection of data pertaining to burn wound infection, invasive device-associated infections such as VAP and CLABSI, and catheter-associated urinary tract infection (CAUTI) will help to estimate the burden and to assess the effectiveness of existing infection control practices.

Standardized definitions of infection and sepsis in burn population, such as CDC's NNIS system, should be used by burn surgeons to identify infections so as to avoid overestimation of infection rates and overuse of antimicrobial agents. The mere presence of an organism does not imply infection. Surface swabs and even quantitative cultures, therefore, do not reliably differentiate colonization from invasion [8]. Histologic examination of a biopsy specimen is the only means of accurately identifying and staging invasive burn wound infection [9].

Routine environmental surveillance cultures are not recommended for BUs except for hydrotherapy and common treatment rooms or during investigation of outbreak in BU.

Infection Prevention and Control Measures

General: Modern burn centers should have a contained perimeter that is designed to minimize the unnecessary traffic of HCP and visitors through the unit. Facilitating BU with all intensive and burn care procedures to be performed within the center itself will avoid transferring patients out and exposing them to risk of cross-contamination. Isolation facilities for individual or cohorts of patients colonized or infected with MRO should be available with separate laminar airflow units. Rate of cross-colonization with resistant organisms in a study of 66 critically ill children with severe burns during five-year period was as low as 3.2 cases per 1,000 patient days in such facility [6].

Infection control practices should be effective in reducing or eliminating endemic pathogenic and/or resistant pathogens and preventing establishment of newly introduced pathogens as predominant nosocomial flora. The infection control program should include the following:

(a) *Barrier techniques*

Open burn wound is a potential source of surrounding environment contamination. As contact is the major mode of transmission of infection, a breach in aseptic precautions can lead to outbreaks in BUs. Strict aseptic techniques should be practiced when handling the open wound. Changing of gloves between patients, wearing impermeable apron or gown, and hand washing before and after using gloves are important. Infrastructure facilities should include enough spacing between beds, provision for enough sinks for washing hands, and proper patient to staff ratio. For improvement in compliance for hand washing, handrubs containing antiseptics should be placed at the footend of each bed.

(b) *Prevention of cross-contamination from inanimate surfaces: disinfection of environment*

Since burn population have extensive openwounds with very high chances of contaminating surrounding environment (bed railings, side table, curtains, mattresses) as well as items such as stethoscope, blood pressure cuff, and thermometer, used on them, secondary transmission to other patients may take place from these heavily organism-laden and frequently touched sites or items. Common treatment rooms are one such source contaminated heavily with MRO which persist for days to weeks, and several outbreaks have been linked to this source. For this reason, environment should be properly cleaned with disinfectants having recommended-use dilution for intended use. A minimum contact time of 1 min should be allowed for efficacy of hospital disinfectants against pathogens. Terminal cleaning of the rooms should be vigorously undertaken before admitting a new patient. Improved surface disinfection can be achieved by educating and training staff.

(c) *Prevention of cross-contamination from convalescent carriers: cohort nursing* Convalescent burn patients may be a reservoir of microorganisms for cross-contamination and infection of burn patients in acute phase. Nursing staff in intensive care unit should not crossover to manage these patients.

(d) *Topical antimicrobial therapy*

Topical antimicrobial application controls the microbial density, thereby decreasing the occurrence of burn wound infection. Resistance to topical antimicrobials in use in a burn care facility may emerge and may be associated with infection outbreaks. Standardized methods should be developed so that clinical microbiology laboratories can perform susceptibility testing for topical agents in use.

(e) *Systemic antimicrobial use in burn patients*

Differentiation of surface colonization from invasive wound infection is crucial to avoid unnecessary systemic antimicrobials in a colonized patient. Colonizing bacteria should never be treated as, firstly, these bacteria cannot be eliminated from the site and recolonize the wound after a probable brief reduction in counts; secondly, not only do these bacteria resurface but also there is a great danger of selecting out MRO. Prior hospitalization and recent receipt of antibiotic are well-known risk factors for acquiring resistant organisms. The development and spread of MRO is a challenge resulting from a combination of both cross-transmission (requiring robust infection control program) and selection of resistant organisms (related to antibiotic misuse and requiring restricted antimicrobial usage). Systemic antibiotic are indicated only as perioperative treatment during excision and grafting [5] and for identified infections of the burn wound, pneumonia, or other systemic infections. Systemic infections should be identified based on clinical signs and culture results, and antimicrobial therapy should be guided by the culture and sensitivity results. Local antibiograms with organism-specific susceptibility data reviewed 6 monthly or at least annually can assist in formulating antibiotic policy of the BU.

(f) *Early excision of wound and grafting*
Early burn wound excision and closure reduces burn wound infection and mortality and also ensures penetration of optimal concentration of the drug up to the surface of viable tissue.

(g) *Surveillance of hospital-associated infections and monitoring of systemic antibiotic use* as described previously

(h) *Care of invasive devices*
Catheters should preferably be placed at a distance from burned areas. Staff should be educated to routinely use handrubs before handling the catheters and on appropriate care of catheters. Need for catheter should be daily reviewed. Antibiotic-impregnated catheters can be used for long-term use to reduce infections. Catheter removal is recommended in the event of CLABSI; alternatively, antibiotic lock therapy has shown great promise in salvaging the infected catheters. Head elevation, daily chest physiotherapy, changing sides, and frequent suctioning are effective in preventing pneumonia in these patients.

(i) *Role of selective decontamination of gut* is unclear in preventing sepsis in the severely burned as contrasting data are available in literature [10, 11]. Further studies are needed to elucidate its usefulness in this population.

Summary

Burn wound invasive infections continue to be the significant cause of morbidity and mortality among burn patients despite advances in wound care and modernization of burn care facility designs. Control of infections due to emerging multidrug-resistant organisms is a major challenge in this population. A good infection control program with well-conducted surveillance activities, topical antimicrobial application, strict isolation or barrier nursing techniques, aggressive disinfection protocols, and appropriate use of empirical antimicrobial therapy guided by laboratory surveillance and routine burn wound cultures is essential to minimize the incidence of systemic infections in severely burned patients.

References

1. http://www.who.int/mediacentre/factsheets/fs365/en/. Accessed 15 May 2013.
2. Taneja N, Emmanuel R, Chari PS, Sharma M. A prospective study of hospital-acquired infections in burn patients at a tertiary care referral centre in North India. Burns. 2004;30(7):665–9.
3. Mayhall CG. The epidemiology of burn wound infections: then and now. Clin Infect Dis. 2003; 37(4):543–50.
4. Shankowsky HA, Callioux LS, Tredget EE. North American survey of hydrotherapy in modern burn care. J Burn Care Rehabil. 1994;15:143–6.
5. Steven EW, Basil AP, Seung HK. Infections in burns. In: Cunha BA, editor. Infectious diseases in critical care medicine. 2nd ed. New York: Informa Healthcare USA; 2007. p. 507–25.
6. Weber JM, Neely AN, Mayhall CG. Burns. In: Carrico R, editor. APIC text of infection control and epidemiology. 3rd ed. Washington, DC: APIC; 2009.
7. Dudeck MA, Horan TC, Peterson KD, Allen-Bridson K, Morrell GC, Pollock DA, Edwards JR. National Healthcare Safety Network (NHSN) report, data summary for 2009, device-associated module. Am J Infect Control. 2011;39(5):349–67.
8. Steer JA, Papini RP, Wilson AP, McGrouther DA, Parkhouse N. Quantitative microbiology in the management of burn patients. Correlation between quantitative and qualitative burn wound biopsy culture and surface alginate swab culture. Burns. 1996;22:173–6.
9. Pruitt Jr BA, McManus AT, Kim SH, Goodwin CW. Burn wound infections: current status. World J Surg. 1998;22:135–45.

10. de la Cal MA, Cerdá E, García-Hierro P, van Saene HK, Gómez-Santos D, Negro E, Lorente JA. Survival benefit in critically ill burned patients receiving decontamination of the digestive tract: a randomized placebo-controlled, double-blind trial. Ann Surg. 2005;241:424–30.
11. Barret JP, Jeschke MG, Herndon DN. Selective decontamination of the digestive tract in severely burned pediatric patients. Burns. 2001; 27:439–45.
12. Mozingo DW, McManus AT, Pruitt BA. Infections of burn wounds. In: Jarvis WR, editor. Bennett & Brachman's Hospital Infections. 5th ed. Philadelphia: Lippincott Williams and Wilkins; 2007. p. 599–610.

Infection Prevention for Procedures in Wards

17

Sushant Wattal and Neeraj Goel

Introduction

While we are recognizing the merits of modern medicine and significance of various guidelines in preventing infections including hospital acquired, it is essential to understand the work dynamics of a public hospital in any city in resource-constrained settings. Many invasive procedures are conducted on the patients on the floor like the following:

1. Peripheral and central venous lines
2. Endotracheal intubation
3. Urinary catheterization
4. Any other invasive bedside procedures

Many hospitals have created a facility in their settings by the name as procedure room where all necessary disinfection precautions are in built with a dedicated as well as trained nursing staff. But a vast majority does not have such facilities, and abovementioned high-risk invasive procedures are conducted in the background of the lack of knowledge and nonavailability of items. This renders following of guidelines difficult. In a public sector hospital, most of the disinfectants are not available and conducting such procedures

is a challenge. The doctor conducting the procedure must have the knowledge of the following:

(a) Firm selection of the site of puncture/catheterization to allow no-touch technique.
(b) Concept of sterility by way of proper surgical scrub and use of sterile gloves and its change just before the procedure that is to be conducted after having prepared the site.
(c) Has the patient earned the procedure?
(d) Monitoring of the devices introduced and most importantly its prompt removal, when not required.

Mostly in a public hospital, items that are often available to conduct the procedures are alcohol swab, soap and water, and sterile gloves. Many facilities are using Savlon or Dettol as a disinfectant. Soaps like Savlon could remove the dirt and organisms physically but are very poor killers of the vegetative forms of organisms, whereas Dettol is notorious to grow organism in it. This leaves us with a strong feeling of lack of knowledge and facilities to perform the abovementioned procedure in day-to-day functioning of a public hospital. Needless to say, hand washing facility by the patient bedside is a distant dream in such public hospitals.

There are a large number of hospital-acquired infections (HAI) worldwide, in part due to neglect of practices to prevent HAI. It has been estimated that more than 1.4 million HAI occur each year with highest prevalence in Eastern Mediterranean and South-East Asia Regions (11.8 % and 10.0 %, respectively) [1]. Direct attributable fallout of these HAI is increased cost,

S. Wattal (✉)
Department of Cardiology, G B Pant Hospital,
New Delhi, India
e-mail: supersinger.sush@gmail.com

N. Goel
Department of Clinical Microbiology,
Sir Ganga Ram Hospital, New Delhi, India

duration of hospitalization, and increase in morbidity and mortality.

To reduce these preventable HAI, certain lacunae need to be overcome. Foremost is to understand the need for reduction of these hospital-acquired infections by the management, formulation of institute-specific evidence-based and outcome-oriented guidelines, and their effective implementation and monitoring. The seemingly daunting task can begin with small, easy, and yet effective steps. Education and constant motivation among the junior health-care givers is critical for implementation of guidelines. It is essential to make a right choice of a disinfectant which is the primary requirement before embarking upon any of the invasive procedures on the patients. Two disinfectants Betadine (10 %) or chlorhexidine (0.5–2 %) can be recommended for skin disinfection and should be wiped adequately after drying by 70 % absolute alcohol before the site can be considered as sterile for the procedure. Simple proper hand hygiene, while performing any medical procedure, is the most pivotal measure to prevent hospital-acquired infection, yet its importance and compliance is most neglected even today. Most of the medical procedures are attempted by the resident doctors in a healthcare setting. Many of them are not formally/adequately trained to do or monitor them as per the standard practices. So it is essential to built in the curriculum of resident doctors training of procedures and its care subsequently. It is a frequent practice to put the urinary bag on the abdomen or the bed of the catheterised patient while shifting which leaves a scope for backflow of urine to the bladder, and this could be the source of cystitis in a febrile neutropenic patient and can even lead to urosepsis, even though there is no firm evidence to it.

The overarching goal of hospital-acquired infections associated with medical devices is to improve the health outcomes by reducing adverse events, and it can also save money for the hospital. We have made an attempt to enlist the internationally accepted and practiced guidelines for prevention of device-related HAI.

Intravasular Catheter Associated Infections

Intravascular catheters (IVC) are important devices in the management of patients in modern-day medical practice, particularly in intensive care units. Although IVC provides easy vascular access, their use is associated with complications like local and systemic infections, catheter-related bloodstream infections (CRBSI), septic thrombophlebitis, endocarditis, and other metastatic infections (e.g., lung abscess, brain abscess, osteomyelitis.). Indwelling catheters are also a frequent source of infection, and CRBSI due to IVC remains as the most important cause of morbidity and mortality worldwide.

The rates of CRBSI in US medical and surgical ICUs are reported from 1.4 to 2.0 per 1,000 catheter days. The higher incidence of CRBSI is reported in resource-poor countries ranging from 1.6 to 44.6 cases per 1,000 catheter days [2]. In India, there is scant published data on CRBSI, but is estimated to be as high as 8.75 per 1,000 catheter days [3]. The higher incidence of CRBSI in resource-poor countries is secondary to the lack of infection control practices. There is growing consensus that CRBSIs are preventable through the use of existing techniques, and health institutes should earnestly device protocols to reduce these preventable nosocomial infections. As an example, the incidence of CRBSI associated with central lines among patients hospitalized in intensive care units (ICUs) in the United States decreased from 3.64 to 1.65 infections per 1,000 central line days between 2001 and 2009 [4].

The following guidelines are recommended by the authors for decreasing IVC-related CRBSI:

I. *Education, training, and staffing* [5, 6]
  1. Educate healthcare personnel who insert and maintain the IVC for the following:
    (a) Indications for intravascular catheter use
    (b) Proper procedures for the insertion
    (c) Maintenance of IVC
  2. Periodically assess knowledge of all personnel for adherence to guidelines in the insertion and maintenance of IVC
  3. Ensure appropriate nursing staff levels in ICUs to minimize the incidence of CRBSIs

II. *Catheter type and site selection* [5, 7–9]
1. Peripheral and midline catheter recommendations:
   (a) In adults, use an upper-extremity site for catheter insertion rather than the lower extremity.
   (b) In pediatric patients, the upper or lower extremities can be used for catheter insertion.
   (c) Avoid the use of steel needles for the administration of fluids and medication which might cause tissue necrosis if extravasation occurs.
   (d) Monitor the catheter sites visually or by palpation through the intact dressing on a regular basis, depending on the clinical situation of individual patients. If patients have tenderness at the insertion site, fever without obvious source, or other manifestations suggesting local or BSI, the dressing should be removed to allow thorough examination of the site.
   (e) Record the operator, date, and time of catheter insertion and removal and dressing changes on a standardized form.
   (f) Do not routinely culture catheter tips.
   (g) Remove peripheral venous catheters if the patient develops signs of phlebitis, infection, or a malfunctioning catheter.
2. Central venous catheters recommendations (CVC):
   (a) Use ultrasound guidance to place CVC (where available) to reduce the number of cannulation attempts and mechanical complications.
   (b) Use a CVC with the minimum number of lumens or ports required for the patient management.
III. *Aseptic precautions during insertion and care of IVC* [5, 10]
1. Observe proper hand hygiene procedures either by washing hands with conventional antiseptic-containing soap and water or with waterless alcohol-based gels or foams.
2. Observe hand hygiene at appropriate time points (before and after palpating catheter insertion sites, as well as before and after inserting, replacing, accessing, repairing, or dressing an intravascular catheter).
3. Use maximum sterile barrier precautions, including a cap, mask, sterile long-sleeve gown, sterile gloves, and head-to-toe sterile body drape.
4. Disinfect clean skin with an appropriate antiseptic before catheter insertion and during dressing changes. Although a 2 % chlorhexidine-based preparation is preferred, tincture of iodine, an iodophor, or 70 % alcohol can be used.
5. Use a 2 % chlorhexidine wash for daily skin cleansing to reduce CRBSI.
IV. *Catheter site dressing regimens* [5, 11]
1. Preferably use sterile gauze with transparent, semipermeable dressing to cover the catheter site to allow daily examination.
2. Change the dressing when it becomes damp, loosened, or visibly soiled.
3. Do not use topical antibiotic ointment or creams at the insertion sites (except when using dialysis catheters) because of their potential to promote fungal infections and antimicrobial resistance.
4. Replace dressings used on short-term CVC sites every 2 days for gauze dressings. Replace dressings used on short-term CVC sites at least every 7 days with transparent dressings, except in those pediatric patients in which the risk for dislodging the catheter may outweigh the benefit of changing the dressing.
V. *Antimicrobial catheters* [5]
1. Use antimicrobial-coated catheters (chlorhexidine/silver sulfadiazine or minocycline/rifampin) if it is expected to remain in place for >5 days, if rates of CRBSI remain above the goal set by the institution after implementing strategies I and III given above.
VI. *Prophylactic antimicrobials* [5]
1. Do not administer intranasal or systemic antimicrobial prophylaxis routinely before

insertion or during use of an intravascular catheter to prevent catheter colonization or BSI.

VII. *Antibiotic lock solutions* [2, 5, 12]

1. Do not routinely use antibiotic lock solutions to prevent CRBSI, as emergence of resistant microorganisms can occur.

2. Use prophylactic antibiotic lock solution only in special circumstances (e.g., in treating a patient with a long-term cuffed or tunneled catheter or port who has a history of multiple CRBSIs despite optimal maximal adherence to aseptic technique).

3. It is prudent to avoid using antibiotics that are commonly used in the therapy of BSIs (such as beta-lactams, vancomycin, quinolones, and aminoglycosides). Minocycline, EDTA, citrate, or ethanol can be used for such therapies.

VIII. *Replacement of catheters and administration sets* [2, 5]

1. Remove any intravascular catheters immediately that are not essential.

2. Replace peripheral venous catheters at least every 72–96 h in adults to prevent phlebitis.

3. Leave peripheral venous catheters in place in children until IV therapy is completed, unless complications (e.g., phlebitis and infiltration) occur.

4. Do not routinely replace central venous or routinely change catheters using guide wires to prevent infection.

5. Use clinical judgment to determine when to replace a catheter that could be a source of infection (e.g., do not routinely replace catheters in patients whose only indication of infection is fever). Do not routinely replace venous catheters in patients who are bacteremic or fungemic if the source of infection is unlikely to be the catheter.

6. Replace any short-term CVC if purulence is observed at the insertion site, which indicates infection.

7. When adherence to aseptic technique cannot be ensured (i.e., when catheters are inserted during a medical emergency), replace all catheters as soon as possible and after no longer than 48 h.

8. Replace continuously used administration sets between 4 and 7 days.

9. Replace tubing used to administer blood, blood products, or fat emulsions within 24 h of initiating and replace tubing used to administer propofol infusions every 6–12 h.

Ventilator-Associated Pneumonia

The term ventilator-associated pneumonia (VAP) refers to pneumonia that arises more than 48–72 h after endotracheal intubation with no clinical evidence suggesting the presence or likely development of pneumonia at the time of intubation [13]. VAP is a complication of intubation and ventilatory support and represents an important health problem that generates great controversy. VAP prolongs ICU length of stay and may increase the risk of death in critically ill patients, but the attributable risk of VAP appears to vary with patient population and causative organism. The incidence of VAP is 3 % per day in the first week, 2 % per day in the second week, and 1 % per day thereafter [14]. The strongest risk factor for VAP is tracheal intubation and occurs in 9–27 % of all intubated patients [13]. In ICU patients, nearly 90 % of episodes of HAP occur during mechanical ventilation. Estimated rate of secondary bacteremia due to VAP is 4–38 % and median crude mortality rate of 41.5 % [14].

Various strategies have been formulated for prevention of VAP [13, 15], which are summarized below:

I. *General prophylaxis* [13, 16]

1. Use effective infection control measures including staff education, compliance with alcohol-based hand disinfection, and isolation to reduce cross-infection with MDR pathogens.

2. Perform surveillance of VAP to identify patients with VAP and calculation of VAP rates (i.e., the number of VAP cases and number of ventilator days for all patients

who are undergoing ventilation and in the population being monitored) and preparation of timely data for infection control.

II. *Strategies to reduce risk of VAP during endotracheal intubation* [13, 15–17]

1. Maintain hand hygiene and adequate barrier precautions during intubation.

2. During laryngoscopy and endotracheal intubation care should be taken to ensure that the sterile tube does not touch external surfaces.

3. Avoid intubation and re-intubation, if possible, as it increases the risk of VAP 6–21-fold.

4. Use noninvasive ventilation, like face mask, wherever possible.

5. Minimize the duration of ventilation, such as improved sedation and early weaning.

6. Avoid nasogastric intubation and prefer orotracheal intubation. Nasogastric intubation is associated with increased risk of sinusitis and VAP.

7. Continuous aspiration of subglottic secretions can reduce the risk of early-onset VAP and should be used, if available.

8. Maintain an endotracheal cuff pressure of at least 20 cm H_2O to prevent leakage of bacterial pathogens around the cuff into the lower respiratory tract.

9. Maintain patients in a semi-recumbent position (30°–45°) rather than supine to prevent aspiration. Though, recent studies show that it is difficult to maintain this position at all the times.

III. *Strategies to minimize contamination of equipment* [15, 18, 19]

1. Use sterile water to rinse reusable respiratory equipment.

2. Remove contaminated condensate from ventilatory circuits and prevent it from entering either the endotracheal tube or inline medication nebulizers. Keep the ventilatory circuit closed during condensate removal.

3. Do not routinely change the ventilator circuit more frequently than 72 h unless visibly soiled or mechanically malfunctioning.

IV. *Strategies to reduce colonization of the aerodigestive tract* [13, 15]

1. Avoid histamine receptor 2 blocking agents and proton pump inhibitors for patients who are not at high risk for developing a stress ulcer or stress gastritis. These agents increase the colonization density of the aerodigestive tract with potentially pathogenic organisms.

2. Perform regular oral care with an antiseptic solution. The optimal frequency for oral care is unresolved.

3. Selective decontamination of the digestive tract with or without systemic antibiotics, though reduces the incidence of ICU-acquired VAP, is an unresolved issue as may select out MDR organisms.

Catheter-Associated Urinary Tract Infections

Urinary tract infections (UTIs) are one of the most common nosocomial infections encountered in healthcare facilities. It is estimated that about 40 % of all nosocomial infections are due to UTIs. Instrumentation (catheterization) is the leading cause of UTIs, the remaining ones are usually associated with some urologic procedures [20]. Apart from infective and noninfective complications of urinary tract, catheter-associated urinary tract infections (CAUTI) are the major cause (20 %) of secondary nosocomial bacteremia, which further increases the associated morbidity and mortality [21].

Introduction of closed sterile urinary drainage in 1950s led to a sharp fall in the rates of CAUTI and is able to prevent 70 % to 85 % of CAUTI [20]. Still the incidence of bacteriuria associated with urethral catheterization with a closed drainage system remains approximately 3 % to 8 % per day. And the overall current rates of CAUTI in healthcare settings range from 0.4 to 6.6 per 1,000 urinary catheter days [20, 22, 23]. Recently, more and more healthcare givers have begun programs to reduce the incidence of CAUTI. The broad guidelines are enumerated here for prevention of CAUTI:

I. *General prophylaxis* [21]
  1. Education and training
    (a) Provide education and training for healthcare personnel regarding techniques and procedures for urinary catheter insertion, maintenance, and removal.
  2. Surveillance
    (a) Consider surveillance for CAUTI when indicated by facility-based risk assessment
    (b) Provide regular feedback of unit-specific CAUTI rates to nursing staff and other appropriate clinical care staff

II. *Appropriate catheter use* [21, 24, 25]
  1. Catheterization should be done only when they are indicated.
    (a) Develop list of appropriate institution specific indications for inserting indwelling urinary catheters.
    (b) Avoid catheters for use in incontinence, for obtaining urine for culture or other diagnostic tests, or for prolonged postoperative duration without appropriate indications.
  2. Remove indwelling catheters as soon as they are no longer required to reduce the risk of catheter-associated bacteriuria.
  3. Consider using alternatives to indwelling urethral catheterization when appropriate.
    (a) Consider condom catheterization as an alternative to indwelling urethral catheters in cooperative male patients without urinary retention or bladder outlet obstruction.
    (b) Consider intermittent catheterization in patients with neurogenic bladder.

III. *Precautions during insertion of catheters* [21, 24]
  1. Appropriate size (smallest bore catheter possible) of catheter should be selected for proper drainage.
  2. Strict asepsis should be maintained during insertion of catheter.
  3. Perform hand hygiene immediately before and after insertion or any manipulation of the catheter device or site. Sterile gloves should be worn after hand washing.
  4. Site should be prepared using chlorhexidine and povidone iodine and should be draped with sterile sheet before catheterization
  5. Apply single-use packet sterile lubricating jelly.
  6. Insert the catheter, taking care that the tip of the catheter should not touch any area outside the urethra.
  7. After insertion, secure the catheter properly to prevent movement and urethral traction.

IV. *Maintenance* [21, 24, 26]
  1. Following aseptic insertion of the urinary catheter, maintain a sterile, continuous, and closed drainage system.
  2. Maintain unobstructed urine flow.
  3. Hang the urine bag to the hook attached to the bed.
  4. Do not let the bag touch the floor.
  5. Avoid raising the level of the urine collection bag to such a height that causes a backflow particularly during transportation of the patient.
  6. Empty the collecting regularly taking precaution to prevent contact of the drainage spigot with the nonsterile collecting container.
  7. Hands should be washed before and after handling the catheter.
  8. Obtain urine aseptically.
    (a) If a small urine sample for culture has to be taken, clean the area over the catheter with alcohol swab and then aspirate with sterile syringe and needle. On removal of the needle, there is no need to seal the site. Sample can also be drawn from the Y connector after cleaning with alcohol.
    (b) Obtain large volume of urine samples for special analysis (not culture) aseptically from the drainage bag.

V. *Prevention of complication of CAUTI* [20, 24, 27]

   1. There is no clear consensus on treatment of asymptomatic bacteriuria in catheterized patients, as its utility has not been evaluated in large-scale clinical trials.

      (a) Routine treatment of asymptomatic bacteriuria may have little clinical benefit and may select out multidrug-resistant organisms.

      (b) Treatment of asymptomatic bacteriuria may have merit in immunocompromised patients and those undergoing urologic operations or surgical procedures involving prosthetic material.

   2. There are no clear cut guidelines on the use of urine cultures (timing and frequency) for the early diagnosis of CAUTI.

   3. There is insufficient data to support use of antimicrobial-coated catheters (silver alloy or antibiotic) to reduce or delay the onset of CA-bacteriuria.

VI. *Important don'ts* [20, 24, 28]

   1. Do not change catheters or drainage bag and tubing routinely unless there is definite evidence of infection and obstruction or when the closed system is compromised.

   2. Do not use systemic antimicrobials prophylaxis to prevent CAUTI in catheterized patients, unless clinical indication exists, e.g., in patients with bacteriuria upon catheter removal post urologic surgery.

   3. Do not clean periurethral area with antiseptics to prevent CAUTI. Routine hygiene (e.g., cleansing of the metal surface during daily bathing or shower) is appropriate.

   4. Do not routinely irrigate catheters with antimicrobials. It may be considered in selected patients who undergo surgical procedures and short-term catheterization to reduce CA-bacteriuria.

   5. Do not add antiseptic or antimicrobial solutions into urinary drainage bags to reduce CAUTI.

Any Other Invasive Bedside Procedure

Besides the above enumerated common procedures done on the floors in any hospital, there are many other procedures like lumber puncture, pleural/ascitic tap, intravascular/muscular injections, bone marrow aspirations, various organ biopsies, and preoperative preparations of the part being conducted by the medical staff on their patients admitted to the wards. The concept of universal precautions for the operator like use of sterile gown, face mask, gloves, and cap remain an essential part of any procedure. However, for the convenience of the reader, an attempt is made below to make some general comments regarding essentials of aseptic precautions.

Before attempting any procedure, make sure that the operator does not have any dermatitis or eczema on his/her hands or in case there is any cut, which is not bandaged appropriately. Make sure that all items required are made available before embarking upon any procedure. Wash your hands with soap and water and dry with disposable towels (do not use a hand drier). Wear an appropriate size of sterile gloves; choose the appropriate site to enable no-touch technique. Prepare the part with a disinfectant like tincture of iodine/2 % chlorhexidine in alcohol; apply in a concentric manner beginning from the site of puncture. Allow three applications to dry and mop in case of iodine with alcohol before the beginning of a procedure. Remove the pair of gloves and replace it with a new pair of sterile gloves to enable handling of the device that is to be used on the patient. It is essential to understand that primarily it is the devices used on the patients in interventions that are the main cause of hospital-acquired infections. Ensure sterile instruments/equipments alone are used on the patient and avoid reuse of a single-use device unless recommended by the healthcare facility where you are working. Unfortunately, mostly undue emphasis is laid on environment to prevent HAI. During the procedure, maintenance of aseptic precautions is warranted so that the patient is not harmed. After having done the procedure, the puncture site needs to be adequately sealed. 10 % povidone iodine/2 % chlorhexidine in alcohol can be applied and not wiped while the dressing is being done. Both 10 % povidone iodine and 2 % chlorhexidine provide residual effect at the site of applications for 3–4 h.

Infections at the phlebotomy sites can be eliminated if all aseptic precautions at the time of procedure are followed in letter and spirit, and moreover, the recommended disinfectant is 10 % povidone iodine or 2 % chlorhexidine in case of children or adults allergic to iodine. Injection abscesses are the ugliest hospital-acquired infections which should not happen. The cause for such abscesses essentially is due to the use of unsterile devices or noncompliance of aseptic precautions. The healthcare worker needs to understand that the human body is studded with loads of colonizing organisms, and once the intact skin of the patient is insulted by any procedure, it gives an opportunity to the opportunistic pathogens to enter and cause infection more so in a sick patient who may be in an immunocompromised state.

Most of the procedures conducted bedside are extremely safe when all precautions are followed. However, current British Guidelines considers the risk of serious complication as about 1 in 1,000 [29].

Further complications of ascitic taps are known to occur in up to 1 % of patients (abdominal hematomas) but are rarely serious or life threatening [30, 31]. More serious complications such as hemoperitoneum or bowel perforation are rare (1/1,000 procedures) [32].

Mostly all bedside procedures are mostly conducted in hospital settings; however, one study found a complication rate of about 20 % when the ascitic tap procedure was done at home [33].

At the same time, serious complications of a properly performed lumbar puncture are extremely rare [34].

Razors should not be used for the preparation of the part for hair removal; instead clippers are recommended. Micro abrasions caused by shaving predisposes to infection instead. Many neurosurgeons even recommend limited clipping of hair that is likely to fall in the line of the incision with

better results with regard to the surgical site infections and is cosmetically more acceptable. Chlorhexidine soap bath preoperatively can reduce the burden of organisms on the body and could be recommended. There is no evidence to suggest the timing for the same whether a night before or the morning of surgery.

References

1. World Health Organization. Prevention of hospital-acquired infections. A practical guide. 2nd ed. Available at: http://www.who.int/csr/resources/publications/whocdscsreph200212.pdf. Accessed 10 June 2013.
2. Chaftari AM, Raad I. Healthcare-associated infections related to use of intravascular devices Inserted for long-term vascular access. In: Mayhall C, editor. Hospital epidemiology and infection control. 4th ed. Philadelphia: Lippincott Williams & Wilkins; 2012. p. 248–57.
3. Parameswaran R, Sherchan JB, Varma DM, Mukhopadhyay C, Vidyasagar S. Intravascular catheter-related infections in an Indian tertiary care hospital. J Infect Dev Ctries. 2011;5(6):452–8.
4. Centers for Disease Control and Prevention (CDC). Vital signs: central line-associated blood stream infections–United States, 2001, 2008, and 2009. MMWR Morb Mortal Wkly Rep. 2011;60.
5. O'Grady NP, Alexander M, Burns LA, Dellinger EP, Garland J, Heard SO, et al. Healthcare Infection Control Practices Advisory Committee. Guidelines for the prevention of intravascular catheter-related infections. Am J Infect Control. 2011;39(4 Suppl 1): S1–34.
6. Warren DK, Zack JE, Cox MJ, Cohen MM, Fraser VJ. An educational intervention to prevent catheter-associated bloodstream infections in a non-teaching community medical center. Crit Care Med. 2003; 31:1959–63.
7. Band JD, Maki DG. Steel needles used for intravenous therapy. Morbidity in patients with hematologic malignancy. Arch Intern Med. 1980;140:31–4.
8. Hind D, Calvert N, McWilliams R, et al. Ultrasonic locating devices for central venous cannulation: meta-analysis. BMJ. 2003;327:361.
9. Clark-Christoff N, Watters VA, Sparks W, Snyder P, Grant JP. Use of triple-lumen subclavian catheters for administration of total parenteral nutrition. JPEN J Parenter Enteral Nutr. 1992;16:403–7.
10. Boyce JM, Pittet D. Guideline for hand hygiene in health-care settings: recommendations of the Healthcare Infection Control Practices Advisory Committee and the HICPAC/SHEA/APIC/IDSA Hand Hygiene Task Force. Infect Control Hosp Epidemiol. 2002;23:S3–40.

11. Madeo M, Martin CR, Turner C, Kirkby V, Thompson DR. A randomized trial comparing Arglaes (a transparent dressing containing silver ions) to Tegaderm (a transparent polyurethane dressing) for dressing peripheral arterial catheters and central vascular catheters. Intensive Crit Care Nurs. 1998;14:187–91.

12. Henrickson KJ, Axtell RA, Hoover SM, et al. Prevention of central venous catheter-related infections and thrombotic events in immunocompromised children by the use of vancomycin/ciprofloxacin/heparin flush solution: a randomized, multicenter, double-blind trial. J Clin Oncol. 2000;18:1269–78.

13. American Thoracic Society; Infectious Diseases Society of America. Guidelines for the management of adults with hospital-acquired, ventilator-associated, and healthcare-associated pneumonia. Am J Respir Crit Care Med. 2005;171(4):388–416.

14. Bergmans DC, Bonten MJ. Healthcare associated Pneumonia. In: Mayhall C, editor. Hospital epidemiology and infection control. 4th ed. Philadelphia: Lippincott Williams & Wilkins; 2012. p. 307–20.

15. Coffin SE, Klompas M, Classen D, Arias KM, Podgorny K, Anderson DJ, et al. Strategies to prevent ventilator-associated pneumonia in acute care hospitals. Infect Control Hosp Epidemiol. 2008;29 Suppl 1:S31–40.

16. Tablan OC, Anderson LJ, Besser R, Bridges C, Hajjeh R, Healthcare Infection Control Practices Advisory Committee, Centers for Disease Control and Prevention. Guidelines for preventing health-care–associated pneumonia, 2003: recommendations of the CDC and the Healthcare Infection Control Practices Advisory Committee. MMWR Recomm Rep. 2004; 53(RR-3):1–36.

17. Craven DE, Steger KA. Nosocomial pneumonia in mechanically ventilated adult patients: epidemiology and prevention in 1996. Semin Respir Infect. 1996; 11:32–53.

18. Craven DE, Goularte TA, Make BJ. Contaminated condensate in mechanical ventilator circuits: a risk factor for nosocomial pneumonia? Am Rev Respir Dis. 1984;129:625–8.

19. Cook D, De Jonghe B, Brochard L, Brun-Buisson C. Influence of airway management on ventilator-associated pneumonia: evidence from randomized trials. JAMA. 1998;279:781–7.

20. Burke PJ, Pombo DJ. Healthcare-associated urinary tract infections. In: Mayhall C, editor. Hospital epidemiology and infection control. 4th ed. Philadelphia: Lippincott Williams & Wilkins; 2012. p. 270–85.

21. Gould CV, Umscheid CA, Agarwal RK, Kuntz G, Pegues DA. Healthcare Infection Control Practices Advisory Committee. Guideline for prevention of catheter-associated urinary tract infections 2009. Infect Control Hosp Epidemiol. 2010;31(4):319–26.

22. Garibaldi RA, Burke JP, Dickman ML, et al. Factors predisposing to bacteriuria during indwelling urethral catheterization. N Engl J Med. 1974;291:215–19.

23. Classen DC, Larsen RA, Burke JP, et al. Prevention of catheter-associated bacteriuria: clinical trial of methods to block three known pathways of infection. Am J Infect Control. 1991;19:136–42.

24. Hooton TM, Bradley SF, Cardenas DD, Colgan R, Geerlings SE, Rice JC, et al. Diagnosis, prevention, and treatment of catheter-associated urinary tract infection in adults: 2009 International Clinical Practice Guidelines from the Infectious Diseases Society of America. Clin Infect Dis. 2010;50(5):625–63.

25. Griffiths R, Fernandez R. Strategies for the removal of short-term indwelling urethral catheters in adults. Cochrane Database Syst Rev. 2007;(2):CD004011.

26. Kunin CM, McCormack RC. Prevention of catheter-induced urinary tract infections by sterile closed drainage. N Engl J Med. 1966;274:1155–61.

27. Schumm K, Lam TB. Types of urethral catheters for management of short-term voiding problems in hospitalised adults. Cochrane Database Syst Rev. 2008; (2):CD004013.

28. Niel-Weise BS, van den Broek PJ. Antibiotic policies for short-term catheter bladder drainage in adults. Cochrane Database Syst Rev. 2005;(3):CD005428.

29. Moore KP, Aithal GP. Guidelines on the management of ascites in cirrhosis. Gut. 2006;55:1–12. doi:10.1136/gut.2006.099580.

30. Runyon BA. Paracentesis of ascites fluid: a safe procedure. Arch Int Med. 1986;146:2259–61.

31. McVay PA, Toy PTCY. Lack of increased bleeding after paracentesis and thoracentesis in patients with mild coagulation abnormalities. Transfusion. 1991;13:164–71.

32. Runyon BA. Management of adult patients with ascites due to cirrhosis. Hepatology. 2004;39:841–56.

33. Gomara Villabona S, Fernandez-Miera M, Sanroma Mendizabal P, et al. Evacuatory paracentesis at home: why not in primary care. Aten Primaria. 1998;22(2):109–11.

34. Sempere AP, Berenguer-Ruiz L, Lezcano-Rodas M, Mira-Berenguer F, Waez M. Lumbar puncture: its indications, contraindications, complications and technique. Revista de neurologia. 2007;45(7):433–6. PMID 17918111.

Printed by Publishers' Graphics LLC
LMO140214.15.17.28